CANCER ETIOLOGY, DIAGNOSIS AND TREATMENTS

PATHOBIOLOGY OF HEPATOCELLULAR CARCINOMA AND CLINICAL IMPACT

CANCER ETIOLOGY, DIAGNOSIS AND TREATMENTS

Additional books in this series can be found on Nova's website under the Series tab.

Additional e-books in this series can be found on Nova's website under the e-books tab.

CANCER ETIOLOGY, DIAGNOSIS AND TREATMENTS

PATHOBIOLOGY OF HEPATOCELLULAR CARCINOMA AND CLINICAL IMPACT

ANTONIO MAZZOCCA
PASQUALE AGOSTI
AND CARLO SABBÀ

New York

Library of Congress Cataloging-in-Publication Data

Library of Congress Control Number: 2016950212
ISBN: 978-1-53610-002-0

Published by Nova Science Publishers, Inc. † New York

Contents

Author Biography

Antonio Mazzocca, MD, PhD, was born in Barletta, Italy in 1965. After graduating from the Medical School of the University of Bari in 1994, he served as a Navy physician (Medical Officer) in the Italian Navy Medical Corps. Following a PhD in Clinical Pathophysiology at the University of Florence Italy, which he finished in 2001, he moved to the USA, where he continued his postdoctoral research at the laboratory of Alex Toker at Harvard Medical School in Boston for the next three years (2001-2004). Working with Professor Toker, he identified a soluble protein named ADAM9-S secreted by hepatic stromal cells, discovered as important for tumor invasion. His research interest has focused on cell and molecular basis of pathogenic mechanisms underlying liver cancer progression, with particular focus on molecules regulating tumor-stromal interactions. He continued his research on factors involved in cancer progression after moving to Vanderbilt University in 2007. Back to Italy, he was appointed as Assistant Professor of Laboratory Medicine at University of Bari School of Medicine and promoted to Associate Professor in Gastroenterology in 2012 (National Scientific Qualification). Here, he continued his work on hepatic cancer and identified lysophosphatidic acid receptor LPAR6, a protein that supports the growth and tumorigenesis of hepatocellular carcinoma. His research on factors promoting liver cancer growth has proven crucial to understanding the development of cancer and designing anti-cancer drugs. He has published several papers and this is his 1st book. He received several Investigator Awards and he is also the Associate Editor of the Journal of Gastrointestinal Cancer and BMC Cancer. (For further reading please also visit http://www.antoniomazzocca.com/).

Pasquale Agosti, MD, was born in Bari, Italy in 1986. He graduated in Medicine and Surgery at the University of Bari in 2012. He is currently geriatric medical resident at the Interdisciplinary Department of Medicine University of Bari School of Medicine. During the last 2 years, while working in the medical management, he began to show interest in the field of medical research, engaging in clinical and experimental research in the field of hepatology.

Carlo Sabbà, MD, PhD, was born in Bari, Italy in 1952. He graduated in Medicine and Surgery at the University of Bari in 1977. From 1978 to 1981 he did a fellowship for the Italian Research Council. From 1981 he began Assistant Professor in Internal Medicine at the University of Bari. From 1980 to 1983, he was "Visiting Professor" in several Universities of France and in 1983 he got the Italian Board in Internal Medicine. In 1987, he earned his PhD in "Pedagogie des sciences de la sanitè," Universitè Bobigny-Paris France. In 1988, he worked as an Assistant Professor at the Ultrasond Unit Rochester University (NY), USA. From 1988 to 1990, he was "Research Fellow" at the Hepatic Hemodynamic Laboratory and Department of Radiology, Ultrasond Section, New Haven, USA. In 1990, he was "Visiting professor" at the Unit of Ultrasonic Angiology-Guy's Hospital London, Great Britain and in 2001, "Visiting Professor"at the HHT center, Yale University CT, USA. From 1999 to 2010, he continued to work at the University of Bari as Associate Professor and then as Full Professor of Internal Medicine. From 2009, he is Chief of the general internal medicine division at General Hospital of Bari, *Policlinico.* Author of 146 scientific international pubblications indexed on Pub med. His main researchs in the field of hepatology concerned Echo-Color Doppler evaluations of portal hypertension in cirrhotic patients and HCC pathobiology.

Abbreviations

ADH3	alcohol dehydrogenase 3
ALDH2	aldehyde dehydrogenase 2
AFP	alpha-fetoprotein
AFP-L3	lens culinaris agglutinin -reactive alpha-fetoprotein
ALPPS	hypertrophy-inducing strategy for staging hepatectomy
ALT	alanine transaminase
Ang-1	angiopoietin 1
AOS	consensus statement from the Asian Oncology Summit 2009
AP	activator protein
APC	adenomatous polyposis coli
ATX	autotaxin
BCLC	Barcelona Clinic Liver Cancer system
BMI	body mass index
BRCA2	breast cancer type 2
CCl4	carbon tetrachloride
CCN1	matricellular protein cysteine-rich protein 61
CD	cluster of differentiation
CIN	chromosomal instability
CK	cytokeratin
CKI	cyclin-dependent kinase inhibitor
CGH	comparative genomic hybridization
CLIP	Cancer of the Liver Italian Program score
COX	cyclooxygenase
CP	Child Pugh score
CTP	Child-Turcotte-Pugh score
CSCs	cancer stem cells

CT	computed tomography
CTGF	connective tissue growth factor
CUPI	Chinese University Prognostic Index
DCP	des gamma carboxy prothrombin
DEN	diethylnitrosamine
DMN	dimethylnitrosamine
DNs	dysplastic nodules
DNMTs	DNA methyltransferases
DWI	diffusion weighted imaging
EASL	European Association for the Study of the Liver
ECM	extracellular matrix
ECOG	Eastern Cooperative Oncology Group performance status test
ELF	enhanced liver fibrosis test
EORTC	European Organisation for Research and Treatment of Cancer
EpCAM	epithelial cell adhesion molecule
EGF	epidermal growth factor
EGFR/ ERBB	epidermal growth factor receptor
ER	estrogen receptor
ET-1	endotelin 1
FAK	focal adhesion kinase
FDA	US Food and Drug Administration
FGF	fibroblast growth factor
FLR	future liver remnant
FLT3	fms related tyrosine kinase 3
GGT	gamma-glutamyl transpeptidase
GPC3	glypican-3
GRB2	growth factor receptor-bound protein 2
GSK	glycogen synthase kinase
GST-M1	glutathione s-transferase mu 1
GST-T1	glutathione s-transferase theta 1
GSTP1	glutathione s-transferase pi 1
GTP	guanosine-5'-triphosphate
HAI	hepatitis activity index
HBV	hepatitis B virus
HBsAg	hepatitis B surface antigen
HCC	hepatocellular carcinoma
HCV	hepatitis C virus
HER	human epidermal growth factor receptor

HGDNs	high-grade dysplastic nodules
HGF	hepatocyte growth factor
HIF-1A	hypoxia-inducible factor 1-alpha
HPCs	hepatic stem cells
HSP-70	*heat shock protein 70*
HURP	hepatoma-up-regulated protein
ICG	indocyanine green
IGF2R	insulin-like growth factor 2 receptor
IFN	interferon
IL	interleukin
JIS	Japan Integrated Staging score
JNK	c-Jun N-terminal kinases
KRT19	keratin 19, type 1
LAK	lymphocytes with recombinant interleukin-2
LCSGJ	Liver Cancer Study Group of Japan
LOH	loss of heterozygosity
LPA	lysophosphatidic acid
LPAR	lysophosphatidic acid receptor
LPC	lysophosphatidylcholine
LRP	lipoprotein receptor-related protein
LTx	liver transplantation
MAPK	*mitogen-activated protein kinases*
MCP-1	monocyte chemotactic protein-1
M-CSF	macrophage colony-stimulating factor
MDCT	multidetector computed tomography
MELD	model for end-stage liver disease score
MFBs	myofibroblasts
MMPs	metalloproteases
mRECIST	modified *Response Evaluation Criteria In Solid Tumors*
MRI	magnetic resonance imaging
mRNA	messenger *ribonucleic acid*
MRNs	macroregenerative nodules
MSCs	mesenchymal stem cells
NAFLD	nonalcoholic fatty liver disease
NASH	nonalcoholic steatohepatitis
NCCN	National Comprehensive Cancer Network
NF-kβ	nuclear factor kappa-light-chain-enhancer of activated B cells
NK	natural killer
NS	nonstructural *protein*

OV-6	oval cell marker antibody
p160ROCK/	
ROCK 1	rho-associated, coiled-coil-containing protein kinase 1
PCNA	proliferating cell nuclear antigen
PCR	polymerase chain reaction
PDGF	platelet derived growth factor
PDGFR	platelet derived growth factor receptor
PEI	percutaneous ethanol injection
PIAF	cisplatin (platinol) with interferon, doxorubicin, and 5-fluorouracil
PI4KII	phosphatidylinositol 4-kinase type 2 alpha
PIVKA-II	vitamin K absence or antagonist-II
PPAR-γ	peroxisome proliferator-activated receptor gamma
PTEN	phosphatase and tensin homolog
PT INR	prothrombin time international normalized ratio
PTMA	prothymosin-alpha
PVE	portal vein embolization
PVT	portal vein thrombosis
RAMP3	receptor activity modifying protein 3
RAN	ras-related nuclear protein
RasGEF	ras guanine nucleotide exchange factors
RASSF1	ras association domain family member 1
RECIST	*Response Evaluation Criteria In Solid Tumors*
RFA	percutaneous radiofrequency ablation
RhoC	ras homolog *gene* family, member C
ROS	reactive oxygen species
SERCA	sarcoplasmic/endoplasmic reticulum calcium ATPase
SERPINE1	serpin peptidase inhibitor, clade E 1
sFRP1	secreted frizzled-related protein 1
SOCS-1	suppressor of cytokine signaling 1
STAT-1	signal transducer and activator of transcription 1
TAF9	TATA box binding protein-associated factor
TEMs	tetraspanin-enriched microdomains
TERC	telomerase RNA component
TGF	transforming growth factor
Th	T helper lymphocytes
TACE	hepatic artery chemoembolization
TIMP	tissue inhibitor inhibitors of metalloproteases
TIN2	TERF1-interacting nuclear factor 2

TNF	tumor necrosis factor
TNM	Tumor, Node, Metastasis system
TRF1-2	telomeric repeat factor 1-2
TTP	tristetrapolin
US	ultrasonography
VEGF	vascular endotelial growth factor
VEGFR	vascular endotelial growth factor receptor
WHO	World Health Organization

Preface

This book describes the pathobiology of hepatocellular carcinoma underlining its clinical impact in terms of diagnosis, prognosis and novel therapeutic management. In Europe, the common background of HCC is generally viral or alcoholic cirrhosis, however, an increasing number of HCCs develops on inflammatory conditions such as NASH or NAFLD related to metabolic syndrome. The process of carcinogenesis in cirrhotic patients is a multistep process ranging from regenerative to dysplastic nodules characterized by specific alterations including genetic or epigenetic abnormalities. In this context, the tumor microenvironment (i.e., immune and inflammatory response and stromal reaction) is crucial for the transition from the dysplastic nodule to HCC. Extracellular matrix proteins, tetraspanins, ADAMs, TGF-β and the lysophosphatidic acid (LPA) signaling axis are just few examples of mediators that will be reviewed in this book as paradigms in the process of HCC development and progression. The growing knowledges in the complex crosstalk between HCC cells and microenvironment and in the signaling pathways involved will make possible novel target therapies and patient outcome improvements.

Introduction to Hepatocellular Carcinoma (HCC)

Hepatocellular carcinoma (HCC) is considered the sixth most common cancer worldwide and the third malignancy as cause of cancer-related death. In the last 30 years, in USA, there has been a significant increase of HCC incidence (which probably reflects HCV incidence) that is still growing. To date, lung, breast, prostate and colorectal cancer are considered the “four big killer” in USA. However, a predictive study shows that HCC will become the third leading cause of cancer-related deaths by 2030 [1]. This may seem surprising considering the predicted reduction of incidence of both HBV and HCV infection, but it is not surprising considering the increased lifespan of chronic HCV patients and the emerging HCC risk factors. What is really changing is the fraction of HCC not related to common risk factors and so the significant increasing incidence of metabolic conditions such as diabetes, obesity and metabolic syndrome could explain HCC increase. HCC will become a very frequent tumor strongly influenced by life style. Accordingly, liver steatosis or NASH can be considered precancerous conditions. Several environmental and biological factors are involved in liver cancer development, but many studies are necessary to understand better its pathobiology. Therefore, aim of this book is to overview most of the actual knowledge about the pathobiology underlying HCC development and progression and how this knowledge may improve the management of HCC patients.

Reference

[1] Lola Rahib, Benjamin D. Smith, Rhonda Aizenberg, Allison B. Rosenzweig, Julie M. Fleshman, Lynn M. Matrisian. 2014. "Projecting Cancer Incidence and Deaths to 2030: The Unexpected Burden of Thyroid, Liver, and Pancreas Cancers in the United States." *Cancer Res* 74:2913-21.

Chapter 1

Pathobiology of HCC: The Role of Risk Factors

The Role of the Known Environmental Risk Factors

Inflammation, regeneration and fibrosis are the three common features of liver cirrhosis, which is the most common background for HCC development. Known factors associated with an increased risk for HCC are hepatitis B or hepatitis C chronic infection, ethanol chronic consumption, non-alcoholic fatty liver disease (NAFLD), nonalcoholic steatohepatitis (NASH), aflatoxin B1 or other food contaminant fungal toxins. Other factors less commonly associated are hereafter listed and include hemochromatosis, primary biliary cirrhosis, Wilson's disease, α1 antitrypsin deficiency, porphyria cutanea tarda, glycogen storage diseases, citrullinemia, tyrosinemia, autoimmune hepatitis and alagille syndrome of infants. Liver cirrhosis is considered a pre-malignant condition, but not all cirrhotic patients have similar cancer risk. For example, cirrhotic patients with older age, male gender, and severity of hepatopathy have an increased risk of developing HCC. Co-infections such as HBV and HCV, HCV and HIV, or HCV plus alcohol greatly increase the cancer risk. Most cases of HCC (about 80%) occur in sub-Saharan Africa or in Eastern Asia. Other high-rate areas include Senegal, Gambia and South Korea. Southern European countries including Italy are medium-rate areas. Also, the incidence of HCC can vary largely among populations living in the same region. For instance, HCC rates are 2 times higher in Asians than in African Americans who live in the USA, which in turn is 2 times higher than those in whites. Differences in the prevalence of major risk factors for liver disease could be the explanation [1]. In almost all populations, males have higher liver cancer rates than females, with the male-to-female sex ratio usually between 2:1 and 4:1. This is probably due to a major exposition of men to risk factors such as hepatitis, alcohol, smoke and increased iron stores. However, according to authors supporting the association between elevated circulating levels of testosterone and increased HCC risk [2], the different exposition to risk factors is not only the unique explanation. Age is also an important risk factor. Indeed, HCC has a peak incidence in the sixty-year age group.

Major risk factors for HCC vary region by region. In most high-risk areas, the dominant risk factors are consumption of aflatoxin and chronic HBV infection, whereas chronic HCV infection is the most important risk factor in Japan, Western Europe and USA.

Chronic HBV infection is the main cause of HCC in sub-Saharan Africa and Asia (largely acquired by maternal-child transmission). Unlike HCV infection where cirrhosis is a necessary step for HCC development, HBV carriers can develop HCC regardless of the intermediate step of cirrhosis. Integration of the HBV viral DNA in human genome can induce chromosomal instability resulting in deletions or insertions. Insertional mutations at specific sites can activate certain genes (i.e. cyclin A and SERCA1) involved in regulation of cell division [3-4]. Additional mechanisms contributing to HBV-mediated hepatocarcinogenesis occur through the expression of viral proteins. For example, the HBx viral protein is able to inactivate the p53 tumor suppressor protein as well as to activate promoter elements and transcription factors including AP-1 and NF-kB, thus influencing the expression of the cell cycle, proliferation or apoptotic genes [5-6].

Aflatoxin B1 is a potent natural liver carcinogen widespread in China, Southeast Asia and sub-Saharan Africa, produced by the fungi *Aspergillus flavus* and *Aspergillus parasiticus,* which contaminate stored rice, peanuts, ground nuts, and maize. After conversion to its exo-8, 9-epoxide, Aflatoxin B1 reacts with guanines in the DNA of hepatocytes and forms adducts and DNA alterations that favor hepatocarcinogenesis. Exposure to aflatoxin B1 is often present with HBV infection, and this increases 5–10–fold the risk for HCC compared to the single risk factor. In this synergistic action, p53 inactivation or mutation seems to be a common event in HBV and aflatoxin-induced HCC.

The major risk factor for developing HCC in Japan, Western Europe, and USA is HCV-related cirrhosis. Liver cirrhosis is an intermediate necessary step from HCV infection to HCC and the risk seems proportional to its severity and duration (Figure 1). In HCV-related cirrhosis, HCC develops at an annual rate of 1% to 4% (also to 7% in Japan) [1]. Although HCV-related carcinogenesis is mediated by chronic inflammation and fibrosis, it has been postulated that HCV infection may induce hepatocarcinogenesis through host-viral protein interactions. The HCV proteins associated with hepatocarcinogenesis include HCV core protein, NS3 and NS5A that have been shown to inhibit post-transcriptional expression of p21WAF1, a relevant cyclin-dependent kinase inhibitor (CKI) [7-9]. The HCV core protein has transcriptional regulating functions on different cellular genes including the proto-oncogene c-myc and is a modulator of the host immune response [10]. Other described mechanisms of carcinogenesis include: i) interaction of HCV core protein with components of the MAPK signaling pathway modulating cell proliferation; ii) NS5A inactivation of p53; iii) inhibition of apoptosis by the E1/E2 HCV proteins. These mechanisms highlight the relevant role of HCV in HCC development and may explain why antiviral therapy is so useful for HCC prevention in patients with HCV-related cirrhosis.

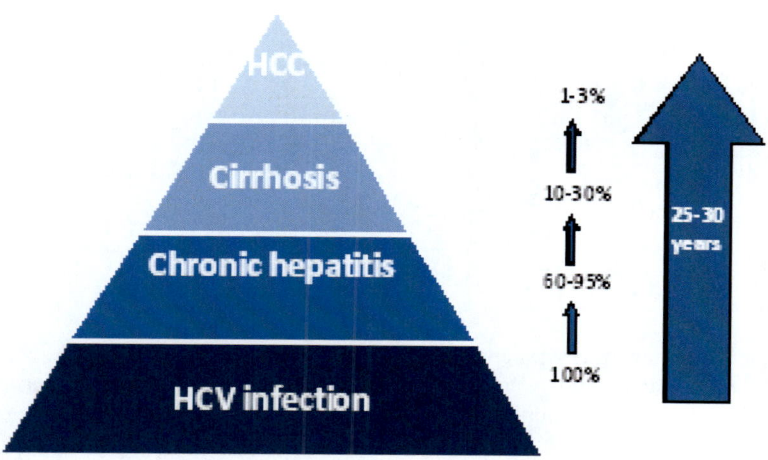

Figure 1. The development of HCC among HCV infected persons is estimated to be from 1 to 3% after 30 years.

Alcohol is associated with the development of cirrhosis, even though a direct carcinogenic effect is not described. Two mechanisms of hepatocarcinogenesis alcohol-related have been proposed: i) the activation of Küpffer cells with release of inflammatory cytokines (TNFα, IL-1) and ii) the oxidative stress, detectable in alcoholic hepatitis as an increase of isoprostane, a marker of lipid peroxidation [11]. Oxidative stress is thought to favor hepatocarcinogenesis in different ways including promotion of fibrosis, oncogenic mutations (i.e. tumor protein p53) and increase of telomere shortening [12-13].

Inflammation, necrosis, regeneration and oxidative stress are the common pathogenic background of HBV-, HCV- and alcohol-induced hepatocarcinogenesis (Figure 2) and a synergistic effect accelerates this process in case of co-morbidity.

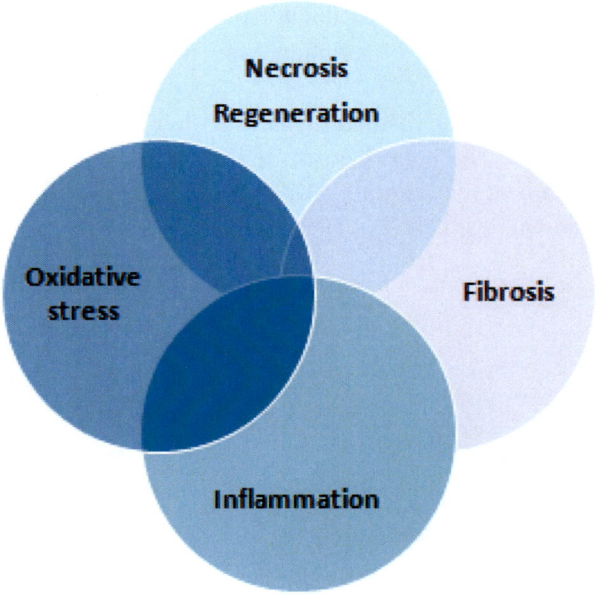

Figure 2. Pathogenic processes representing a common background for HCC development. Inflammation, necrosis, regeneration, fibrosis and oxidative stress are the common pathogenic background of HBV-, HCV- and alcohol-induced hepatocarcinogenesis.

Emerging Risk Factors

Alcohol or viral infections are not the only known environmental risk factors for HCC. An increasing number of HCCs develop on inflammatory conditions such as NASH (nonalcoholic steatohepatitis) or NAFLD (nonalcoholic fatty liver disease) related to metabolic syndrome. For example,

HCC patients with the so-called *cryptogenic cirrhosis* disclose clinical and demographic features suggestive of NASH (predominance of women, diabetes, and obesity) as reported in several studies [14-15].

NAFLD is a condition not necessary associated to NASH. Furthermore, increased levels of steatosis have been associated with more severe necroinflammatory activity, and steatosis itself could be considered an indicator of fibrosis progression [16]. A large number of evidences indicate that the common pathobiological background of these "metabolic-related HCCs" may be insulin-resistance, which has been proposed as an emerging risk factor for HCC along with diabetes and obesity [15]. In a prospective cohort study of more than 900,000 individuals in the USA, liver cancer mortality rates were 5 times greater among men with the greatest body mass index (BMI range: 35–40) compared with those with a normal BMI [17]. Smoking has a weak effect in HCC, probably with a higher risk among women, whereas coffee drinking has been associated with reduced insulin levels, reduced risk for type 2 diabetes and reduced risk of HCC with a dose-dependent effect. In a case-control study odd ratios (OR) were 0.8 for 1-2 cups/day, 0.4 for 3-4 cups/day and 0.3 for coffee dayly consumpion of 5 or more cups [18]. Nuclear estrogen receptors are increased in patients with HCC suggesting a hormonal responsiveness of this malignancy and oral contraceptive abuse has been related to HCC. Finally, the genetic background may have a role in liver cancer development. Indeed, an interesting study has shown a significant increase in cirrhosis prevalence among first-degree relatives of cirrhotic patients, particularly with HCV-related cirrhosis [19]. Similarly, another study reported familial clustering for NAFLD [20]. Several gene polymorphisms have been studied in this field of clinical investigation. Most of these studies have examined polymorphisms in genes involved in detoxification (cytochrome P-450s, N-acetyl transferases, and glutathione S-transferases), inflammation, carcinogenesis (DNA repair i.e. XRCC1), or modulation of the biological effects of alcohol or aflatoxin exposure or other known risk factors (e.g. ADH3, ALDH2, EPHX1). However, these genetic epidemiology studies have produced equivocal results. This lack of reproducibility could be explained considering that individual genes could have only small effects on cancer development because of the stronger influences of environmental risk factors and polygenic effects. Other factors that make all more difficult include differences in the relative distribution of alleles (e.g. among different racial groups) and variabilility in genetic penetrance. A recent study reported a significant association between an epidermal growth factor (EGF) gene polymorphism and increased HCC risk

[21]. Another remarkable study evaluated the effect of the dual-deletion GST polymorphisms GST-M1 and GST-T1, two of the most studied polymorphysms for HCC at the moment that could induce a small excess risk [22]. However, further studies with larger samples including different populations are necessary to better understand the role of both polymorphisms and the crucial crosstalk between genes and environment.

Table 1. Risk factors of hepatocellular carcinoma. The most common risk factors for HCC are listed in the table and include liver cirrhosis, HBV-HCV chronic infections, ethanol chronic consumption, NASH/NAFLD, aflatoxin B1 or other fungal toxins. However, in recent years emerging risk factors have been proposed including insuline-resistance, metabolic syndrome, obesity, diabetes, and gene polymorphisms

Common risk factors	Less common risk factors	Emerging risk factors	Variables
Liver cirrhosis	Hemochromatosis	Insuline-resistance	Sex
HBV-HCV chronic infections	Primary biliary cirrhosis	Metabolic syndrome	Age
Ethanol chronic consumption	Wilson's disease	Obesity	Geographic region
NASH/NAFLD	α1 antitrypsin deficiency	Diabetes	Comorbidity
Aflatoxin B1/ fungal toxins	Porphyria cutanea tarda	Gene polymorphisms	
	Glicogen storage diseases		
	Citrullinemia		
	Tyrosinemia		
	Autoimmune hepatitis		
	Alagille syndrome of infants		

References

[1] El-Serag HB, Rudolph KL. 2007. "Hepatocellular Carcinoma: Epidemiology and Molecular Carcinogenesis." *Gastroenterology* 132: 2557-76.

[2] Yu MW, Chen CJ. 1993. "Elevated serum testosterone levels and risk of hepatocellular carcinoma." *Cancer Res* 53:790-4.

[3] Wang J, Chenivesse X, Henglein B, Bréchot C. 1990. "Hepatitis B virus integration in a cyclin A gene in a hepatocellular carcinoma." *Nature* 343:555-7.

[4] Chami M, Gozuacik D, Saigo K, Capiod T, Falson P, Lecoeur H, Urashima T, Beckmann J, Gougeon ML, Claret M, le Maire M, Bréchot C, Paterlini-Bréchot P. 2000. "Hepatitis B virus related insertional mutagenesis implicates SERCA1 gene in the control of apoptosis." *Oncogene* 19:2877-86.

[5] Chirillo P, Falco M, Puri PL, Artini M, Balsano C, Levrero M, Natoli G. 1996. "Hepatitis B virus pX activates NF-kappa B-dependent transcription through a Raf-independent pathway." *J Virol* 70:641-6.

[6] Henkler F, Lopes AR, Jones M, Koshy R. 1998. "Erk-independent partial activation of AP-1 sites by the hepatitis B virus HBx protein." *J Gen Virol* 79: 2737-42.

[7] Kwun HJ, Jung EY, Ahn JY, Lee MN, Jang KL. 2001. "p53-dependent transcriptional repression of p21(waf1) by hepatitis C virus NS3." *J Gen Virol* 82:2235-41.

[8] Ghosh AK, Steele R, Meyer K, Ray R, Ray RB. 1999. "Hepatitis C virus NS5A protein modulates cell cycle regulatory genes and promotes cell growth." *J Gen Virol* 80:1179-83.

[9] Lee MN, Jung EY, Kwun HJ, Jun HK, Yu DY, Choi YH, Jang KL. 2002. "Hepatitis C virus core protein represses the p21 promoter through inhibition of a TGF-beta pathway." *J Gen Virol* 83:2145-51.

[10] Ray RB, Lagging LM, Meyer K, Steele R, Ray R. 1995. "Transcriptional regulation of cellular and viral promoters by the hepatitis C virus core protein." *Virus Res* 37:209-20.

[11] McClain CJ, Hill DB, Song Z, Deaciuc I, Barve S. 2002. "Monocyte activation in alcoholic liver disease." *Alcohol* 27:53–61.

[12] Marrogi AJ, Khan MA, van Gijssel HE, Welsh JA, Rahim H, Demetris AJ, Kowdley KV, Hussain SP, Nair J, Bartsch H, Okby N, Poirier MC, Ishak KG, Harris CC. 2001. "Oxidative stress and p53 mutations in the

carcinogenesis of iron overload-associated hepatocellular carcinoma." *J Natl Cancer Inst* 93:1652-5.

[13] Kurz DJ, Decary S, Hong Y, Trivier E, Akhmedov A, Erusalimsky JD. 2004. "Chronic oxidative stress compromises telomere integrity and accelerates the onset of senescence in human endothelial cells." *J Cell Sci* 117:2417-26.

[14] Bugianesi E, Leone N, Vanni E, Marchesini G, Brunello F, Carucci P, Musso A, De Paolis P, Capussotti L, Salizzoni M, Rizzetto M. 2002. "Expanding the natural history of nonalcoholic steatohepatitis: from cryptogenic cirrhosis to hepatocellular carcinoma." *Gastroenterology* 123:134-40.

[15] Regimbeau JM, Colombat M, Mognol P, Durand F, Abdalla E, Degott C, Degos F, Farges O, Belghiti J. 2004. "Obesity and diabetes as a risk factor for hepatocellular carcinoma." *Liver Transpl* 10:S69–73.

[16] Adinolfi LE, Gambardella M, Andreana A, Tripodi MF, Utili R, Ruggiero G. 2001. "Steatosis accelerates the progression of liver damage of chronic hepatitis C patients and correlates with specific HCV genotype and visceral obesity." *Hepatology* 33:1358-64.

[17] Calle EE, Rodriguez C, Walker-Thurmond K, Thun MJ. 2003. "Overweight, obesity, and mortality from cancer in a prospectively studied cohort of U.S. adults." *N Engl J Med* 348:1625-38.

[18] Gelatti U, Covolo L, Franceschini M, Pirali F, Tagger A, Ribero ML, Trevisi P, Martelli C, Nardi G, Donato F; Brescia HCC Study Group. 2005. "Coffee consumption reduces the risk of hepatocellular carcinoma independently of its aetiology: a case-control study." *J Hepatol* 42:528-34.

[19] Pagliaro L, Pasta L, D'Amico G, Madonia S, Pietrosi G. 2002. "Familial clustering of (mostly) HCV-related cirrhosis. A case-control study." *J Hepatol* 37:762-6.

[20] Abdelmalek MF, Liu C, Shuster J, Nelson DR, Asal NR. 2006. "Familial aggregation of insulin resistance in first-degree relatives of patients with nonalcoholic fatty liver disease." *Clin Gastroenterol Hepatol* 4:1162-9.

[21] Tanabe KK, Lemoine A, Finkelstein DM, Kawasaki H, Fujii T, Chung RT, Lauwers GY, Kulu Y, Muzikansky A, Kuruppu D, Lanuti M, Goodwin JM, Azoulay D,Fuchs BC. 2008. "Epidermal growth factor gene functional polymorphism and the risk of hepatocellular carcinoma in patients with cirrhosis." *JAMA* 299:53-60.

[22] White DL, Li D, Nurgalieva Z, El-Serag HB. 2008. "Genetic variants of glutathione S-transferase as possible risk factors for hepatocellular carcinoma: a HuGE systematic review and meta-analysis." *Am J Epidemiol* 167:377-89.

Chapter 2

Natural History of HCC

Epidemiological studies have largely shown that hepatocarcinogenesis is strongly related to chronic liver disease. This could be explained considering that cancer development requires several steps leading to the acquisition of cellular and molecular alterations necessary for cell transformation. Although the frequency of replication errors is low in HCC, there is a high prevalence of chromosome abnormalities. HCC natural history has been conventionally divided into three distinct phases: "molecular," "preclinical" and "clinical" [1].

From Molecular to Clinical Phase

The molecular phase includes the cytoplasmic and nuclear alterations. In the preclinical phase, tumor is too small to be detected with the imaging techniques, and this precedes a second period in which tumor is detectable but still asymptomatic. HCC usually becomes symptomatic when it reaches 4.5–8 cm (clinical phase). As regards the molecular phase, it is well known that cell proliferation at the time of carcinogen exposure is a necessary step for "consolidation" of the genotoxic injury into a heritable form. To better study this crucial step, many models of liver cancer utilize a brief exposure to a specific carcinogen with known genotoxic effects during the hepatocellular proliferative state or shortly after a partial hepatectomy or during the postnatal growth phase. In the liver, the identity of the generating HCC cells is quite problematic. Cells that have been proposed susceptible to neoplastic transformation are not only hepatocytes or colangiocites but also hepatic progenitor cells (HPCs)/oval cells and the "non-descript periductular cells" that may be of bone marrow origin and responsive to periportal insult. This may explain the high heterogeneity of HCC since origin and has a clinical relevant impact considering that all these fourline cells would be considered therapeutic cell targets. Oval cells/HPCs are considered bipotent and can generate both hepatocytes and cholangiocytes. Many evidences are suggestive for an origin from a bipotential progenitor: i) oval cell activation accompanies chronic liver diseases and precedes liver cancer; ii) oval cells can be infected by HBV; iii) an admixture of mature cells, cells characterized by an intermediate phenotype between HPCs and malignant hepatocytes or small oval-shaped HPC-like cells expressing OV-6, CK7, CK19 and chromogranin-A has been demonstrated in many liver neoplasms; iv) cells with an HPC phenotype have also been demonstrated in hepatoblastoma and in a relatively rare subset of hepatic malignancies with the coexistence of an HCC and a cholangiocarcinoma components. The relevant role of oval cells in hepatocarcinogenesis was also demonstrated by Dumble et al. who isolated oval cells from p53-null mice and showed that these cells generated HCCs when transplantated into athymic nude mice [2]. Another interesting observation supporting this idea is that cancer formation is reduced when oval cell expansion is inhibited by the tyrosine-kinase inhibitor imatinib mesylate in a choline-deficient diet mouse model [3]. Although it is commonly believed that only a small minority of HCCs derived from the mature hepatocytes, the well-established role of mature hepatocytes in HCC hystogenesis has been described in several mouse models. In one of these studies, Craddock and coworkers demonstrated that, in the mouse liver, the carcinogenic effect of dimethylnitrosamine (DEN) could be exerted only if administration occurred shortly after a partial hepatectomy, particularly after 1 day when 30–40% of hepatocytes are in S phase. Instead, no carcinogenic effect was noticed if the same dose of the same compound was administred to normal adult rats, thus indicating that hepatocytes are the cancer-generating elements in this model [4]. In another mouse model in which HCC generated from hepatocytes after diethylnitrosamine (DEN) exposure, the investigators showed the presence of α-fetoprotein (AFP)-positive hepatocytes, followed by AFP-positive foci or frank AFP-positive HCC tumors, but only a modest amount of oval cell proliferation was observed [5]. In another study, to demonstrate a clonal origin of HCC from mature hepatocytes, the authors marked hepatocytes with β-galactosidase at 1 day after partial hepatectomy and then administrated 2-acetylaminofluorene which led to formation of pre-neoplastic foci, some of which with β-galactosidase-expressing cells directly descended from hepatocytes [6]. As mentioned above, studies regarding the origin of cancer cells in liver cancer have reported contrasting results.

From Macroregenerative to Dysplastic Nodules

Usually the development of HCC requires 10 years from the diagnosis of cirrhosis and 30 years from HCV infection whereas the estimated time to trigger HBV-related carcinogenesis is less predictable [1]. In a cirrhotic liver, HCC can develop from macroregenerative nodules (MRNs) (type of carcinogenesis "nodule in nodule"). However, most HCCs develop in areas of cell dysplasia outside MRNs (*de novo* carcinogenesis) (Figure 3). More than one-third of HCCs appear as multiple nodules that is thought to be the result of intrahepatic metastases from a primary focus or the development of synchronous tumors, frequently HBV-related. The MRNs are detectable in 25% of cirrhotic livers and, according to their size (diameter: 1–2 cm) and tissue texture, are normally distinguishable from the surrounding liver. They are hypovascular with a histological structure similar to that of cirrhotic nodules, but with increased cell proliferation. They usually appear hypoechoic on ultrasonography, however, a hyperechoic aspect can be observed, more often in high-grade dysplastic nodules (HGDNs). The MRNs may present as different lesions with various degrees of atypia/dysplasia. For example, in a 33 months follow-up, Borzio et al. observed a transformation rate towards HCC in 22% of large regenerative nodules, 25% of lowgrade dysplastic nodules and 63% of HGDNs, whereas 15% of the MRNs disappeared during follow-up (87% were large regenerative nodules/low-grade dysplastic nodules) [7]. Dysplastic nodules (DNs) are precancerous lesions with abnormal cytological features including clear cell changes, nuclear crowding and increased thickening of the trabeculae. Microsatellite instability at identical loci and identical allelic mutations have been described in DNs and adjacent HCCs, indicating that HCCs often arise as clonal proliferation of DNs. Japanese authors have subclassified minute HCCs ($\leq$ 2 cm in diameter), which are usually well differentiated, as "indistinctly" and "distinctly" nodular according to the macroscopic feature. Indistinctly nodular HCCs are well-detectable nodular lesions on ultrasonography but indistinct at surgical examination. Histologically, they are very well differentiated tumors, with a hypovascular imaging pattern and lower degree of malignancy. Distinctly nodular HCCs are usually easily identifiable at surgical inspection, moderately differentiated, with a pseudocapsule, hypervascular pattern and a frequent microvascular portal invasion (up to 22%) [8]. HGDN may be difficult to distinguish from well-differentiated HCC, particularly from the "indistinctly nodular" type. Carcinoma cell invasion of portal tracts inside the neoplastic nodules is considered as the hallmark of HCC for Japanese pathologists [9]. As tumor growth progresses, HCC blood supply becomes more dependent on newly formed arterial vessels (neoangiogenesis) and proportionally less dependent on the portal contribution. At the same time, sinusoid-like blood spaces go through a process of capillarization. The risk of microvascular invasion in HCC with expansive growth increases with tumor size and dedifferentiation. Different modes of tumor growth have been described. The "linear" one is constant over time. The "hyperbolic" is initially slow with a subsequent increase, whereas the "parabolic" one declines over time. Some authors described for small HCCs two different growth models, the Gompertzian one, in which the earlier exponential growth decreases during tumor size increasining, and the rapid exponential one. Considering a mean volume doubling time of 204 ± 132 days and according to the Gompertzian type of growth, a 1 cm diameter tumor takes about 150 months to grow beyond 5 cm. According to the exponential model, that nodule, to grow beyond 5 cm, takes only about 48 months [10]. Therefore HCC natural history is characterized by a great heterogeneity and reflects the complexity of its pathobiology.

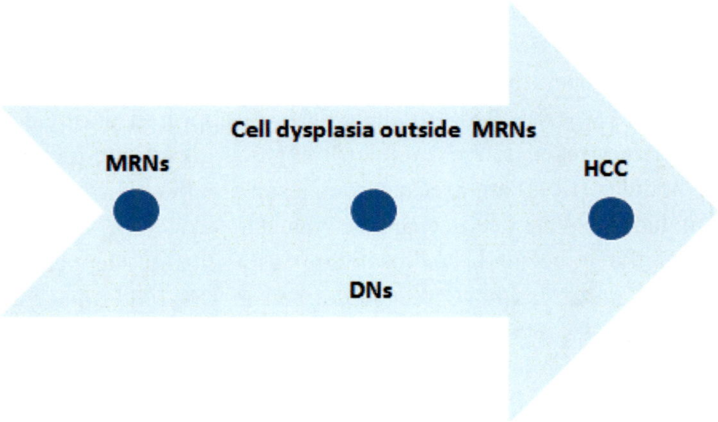

Figure 3. Hepatocarcinogenesis in the cirrhotic liver. In cirrhotic liver, HCC can develop from dysplastic nodules (DNs) that origin from macroregenerative nodules (MRNs) the socalled "*nodule in nodule*" carcinogenesis. However, most HCCs develop from areas of cell dysplasia outside MRNs ("*de novo*" carcinogenesis).

References

[1] Trevisani F, Cantarini MC, Wands JR, Bernardi M. 2008. "Recent advances in the natural history of hepatocellular carcinoma." *Carcinogenesis* 29:1299-305.

[2] Dumble ML, Croager EJ, Yeoh GC, Quail EA. 2002. "Generation and characterization of p53 null transformed hepatic progenitor cells: oval cells give rise to hepatocellular carcinoma." *Carcinogenesis* 23:435-45.

[3] Knight B, Tirnitz-Parker JE, Olynyk JK. 2008. "C-kit inhibition by imatinib mesylate attenuates progenitor cell expansion and inhibits liver tumor formation in mice." *Gastroenterology* 135:969-79,979.

[4] Craddock VM. 1975. "Effect of a single treatment with the alkylating carcinogens dimethynitrosamine, diethylnitrosamine and methylmethane -sulphonate, on liver regenerating after partial hepatectomy. I. Test for induction of liver carcinomas." *Chem Biol Interact* 10:313-21.

[5] Sell S. 2004. "Stem cell origin of cancer and differentiation therapy." *Crit Rev Oncol Hematol* 51:1-28.

[6] Gournay J, Auvigne I, Pichard V, Ligeza C, Bralet MP, Ferry N. 2002. "In vivo cell lineage analysis during chemical hepatocarcinogenesis in rats using retroviral-mediated genetransfer: evidence for dedifferentiation of mature hepatocytes." *Lab Invest* 82:781-8.

[7] Borzio M, Fargion S, Borzio F, Fracanzani AL, Croce AM, Stroffolini T, Oldani S, Cotichini R, Roncalli M. 2003. "Impact of large regenerative, low grade and high grade dysplastic nodules in hepatocellular carcinoma development." *J Hepatol* 39:208-14.

[8] Nakashima O, Sugihara S, Kage M, Kojiro M. 1995. "Pathomorphologic characteristics of small hepatocellular carcinoma: a special reference to small hepatocellular carcinoma with indistinct margins." *Hepatology* 22:101-5.

[9] Tomizawa M, Kondo F, Kondo Y. 1995. "Growth patterns and interstitial invasion of small hepatocellular carcinoma." *Pathol Int* 45:352-8.

[10] Cheng SJ, Freeman RB Jr, Wong JB. 2002. "Predicting the probability of progression-free survival in patients with small hepatocellular carcinoma." *Liver Transpl* 8:323-8.

Chapter 3

Pathobiology of HCC: The Role of Genetic and Epigenetic Factors

Carcinogenesis is considered a stepwise process in which accumulation of chromosomal, genetic and epigenetic abnormalities is necessary to drive cell transformation.

Chromosomal Abnormalities

Recurrent chromosome alterations (i.e., loss of 4q, 8p, 16q, 17p, 13q, 6q and 1p, and gain of 8q, 1q, 6p and 17q) have been revealed by CGH in human HCC [1].

Chromosomal Instability (CIN) emerges at an early stage and accumulates during hepatocarcinogenesis. Complete destruction of telomeres, that is already detectable in preneoplastic hepatocytes, results in chromosomes with "sticky ends" analogous to double-strand breaks producing mitotic non-disjunction. The result of this process is aneuploidy, a common cytogenetic feature in HCC. For example, Aurora kinase A and its target hepatoma up-regulated protein (HURP) are overexpressed in HCC among the genes and proteins involved in chromosome segregation [2]. Furthermore, the spindle-assembly checkpoint is defective in human HCC cell lines as shown by the lack of accumulation of cells in metaphase following treatment with nocodazole or colcemid that normally arrest the cells at metaphase. Mutations in p53, p38, BRCA2 and cohesin are possibly involved [3]. Genome-wide micro-array analysis has been recently employed to study the molecular expression profiles of the different stages of hepatocarcinogenesis to identify a possible "molecular signature" in different steps from dysplastic nodules to HCC. For example, low-grade DNs and MRNs did not show allelic losses on 8p and gains of 1q, as in high-grade DNs and HCCs. Loss of heterozygosity (LOH) at 1p (1p36-p34) or in M6F/IGF2R is an early event in hepatocarcinogenesis [4]. In particular, loss of heterozygosity in the insulin-like growth factor-2 receptor (IGF-2R) locus occurs in more than 60% of dysplastic nodules and HCCs and could cooperate with IGF2 overexpression [5].

Another chromosomal abnormality observed in cirrhosis and in early steps of hepatocarcinogenesis is telomere shortening. In chronic liver diseases, acceleration of telomere shortening occurs and often correlates with fibrosis progression. When telomeres are next to a critical short length, uncapping of chromosomes induces signals that lead to senescence or apoptosis. However, telomere dysfunction can activate DNA repair pathways leading to fused chromosomes, as well as chromosomes breakage during cell cycle perpetuating chromosomal abnormalities in the daughter cells. A gradual shortening of telomere during hepatocarcinogenesis from low grade DNs to high grade DNs has been observed and in the latest, telomere shortening was comparable to HCCs. More than 90% of human HCCs display an activation of telomerase and up-regulation of telomerase reverse transcriptase can be considered a marker of human HCC. In line with this evidence, amplification of the gene that encodes the telomerase RNA component (TERC) and the allelic loss of a region (10p) that encodes a telomerase repressor in HCC have been reported. Oh et al. observed that the expression of the telomere-binding proteins (TRF1, TRF2, TIN2 mRNA) increased in cirrhosis and DNs and that this increase was even more significant in HCCs [6]. In addition, they observed that the telomere lengths were inversely associated with the mRNA level of these genes. Interestingly, studies in TERC null mice showed that telomere dysfunction increased the initiation of HCC, whereas the absence of telomerase activity impaired cancer progression [7]. Therefore, a model wherein telomere shortening drives chromosomal instability and cancer-promoting lesions during early stages of hepatocarcinogenesis has been proposed. However, re-activation of telomerase is required for malignant progression and this sustains cancer cell survival [8]. In addition, telomere reduction occurring in carcinoma-associated fibroblasts (CAFs) enhances secretion of proinflammatory proteins and this might contribute to the creation of a cirrhotic microenvironment [9]. Another area of investigation is the role of telomere shortening and hepatocellular senescence in the loss of replicative reserve during cirrhosis. It is known that telomere dysfunction induces p21-dependent checkpoints that can limit longevity in mice [10] and that upregulation of p21 expression is frequently observed in human chronic liver disease [11].

Genetic Abnormalities

It is commonly believed that development and progression of cancers are accompanied by complex gene alterations. However, in HCC, gene mutations are less frequent when compared with other cancers and, since the "preneoplastic phase" (i.e., chronic hepatitis and cirrhosis) occurs, epigenetic alterations without changes in the genes structure are observed. In HCC, the most frequently mutated genes are p53 and β-catenin and it has been proposed that tumors harboring p53 and β-catenin mutation might arise from two independent pathways. To this purpose, two groups of HCC can be distinguished, one demonstrating chromosome stability, β-catenin mutation and chromosome 8p losses, and the second one showing chromosomal instability, frequent allelic losses on chromosomes 1p, 4q, 6q, 9p, 13q, 16p, 16q and 17p and mutations of p53 and Axin1 genes [12]. The cDNA micro-array has been used to compare the gene expression profiles between human HCCs and the non-tumorous liver tissues from the same patients or from normal livers. Interestingly, "proliferation cluster" including expression of genes involved in cell proliferation is increased in HCC samples and, additionally, most genes expressed at lower levels in HCC are genes specifically expressed in differentiated hepatocytes [13]. These observations suggest that upregulation of proliferation-associated genes have a relevant role in hepatocarcinogenesis. However, cancer cell dedifferentiation occurring during HCC progression may be associated with downregulated liver-specific genes [14]. Several studies have examined whether specific genomic alterations are related to exposition to specific risk factors. In this field cDNA micro-arrays have been successfully used to compare the gene expression profiles between HCC from different etiologies, identifying several specific loci. For example, HBV-related HCCs exhibit a more intense genetic instability with several chromosome changes with more frequent (40%) losses at 4q, 16q and 17p (including the p53 region) and gains in 8q and 20q. These HCCs are observed more frequently in livers with no underlying cirrhosis, suggesting that genetic alterations could induce neoplastic transformation without the cooperation of environmental factors such as cytokines or other signals produced from a fibrotic/cirrhotic background. By contrast, non-HBV related HCCs present less instability, but more frequently display β-catenin mutations and the wnt pathway activation [4]. Furthermore, it has been proposed that certain chromosomal abnormalities or gene mutations could be characteristic for a specific stage of carcinogenesis, ranging from dysplastic lesions to earlier or advanced HCCs. For example, different genes have been related to tumor progression (SOCS-1, PEG10) or metastasis (nm23-H1, osteopontin, KAI1) [4]. Overall, oncogenic pathways activation in HCC is more heterogeneous than other cancers, probably because oncogene activation may occur in the late-stage of human hepatocarcinogenesis as a consequence of chromosomal instability induced by telomere shortening and checkpoint dysfunction.

Some of the most studied gene mutations in HCC are listed hereafter.

p53 and p16/Rb Checkpoints

The activation of the cell cycle checkpoints is crucial in hepatocyte proliferation during cirrhosis and its abrogation is one of the hallmarks of liver carcinogenesis. One of the relevant checkpoints involved in HCC is p53 protein, by limiting cell survival and inducing cell-cycle arrest in response to telomere shortening and oncogene activation, although it is not yet clear whether p53 mutation contributes to cancer initiation, progression or both. In one study using an HBx transgenic mouse model, investigators noticed that functional inactivation of p53 by HBx through its sequestration to the cytoplasm was documented in HCCs but not in initial altered foci [15]. In addition, p53 overexpression was more frequently seen in larger and poor differentiated tumors, suggestive of a late event in HCC progression. On the contrary, in aflatoxin B1-related HCC, p53 mutation might have a role in initiation, but cooperating events are necessary, as demonstrated with the observation that p53 mutant mice do not show an HCC-prone phenotype. This could mean that p53 mutation could have a relevant role in either HCC initiation or progression, according to context differences. In aflatoxin context, as over mentioned, it might have a role in cancer initiation; however in the context of other etiologies as those involved in regeneration, oxidative stress and telomere erosion, p53 suppression could be an important mediator of HCC progression by amplifying cell proliferation and chromosomal instability. Loss of p53 checkpoint function is believed to amplify the number of hepatocytes with chromosomal instability at the stage of cirrhosis [16]. In agreement with this observation, expression of p21, a downstream target in p53 pathway, is increased during cirrhosis and absent in HCC [17]. Mutations in the p53 gene occur more frequently in aflatoxin-induced HCC (50%) than others (20%–40%) [16]. What is also really interesting is the synergistic effect of two or more known risk factors on HCC initiation and progression mediated by p53 mutations. For example, HBsAg transgenic mice have a prone condition to form HCC that is accelerated when combined with aflatoxin B1 administration and the p53ser246 allele, which represents the aflatoxin B1 exposure-related p53 mutation in HCC [18]. In a similar manner, in HBsAg mice heterozygous for a p53 null allele treated with aflatoxin, an increase cancer progression has been demonstrated [19].

p16/Rb is another important cell-cycle checkpoint that is altered in HCC in more than 80% of cases. Increased expression of p16 is detected in liver cirrhosis. However, p16 expression is diminished in HCC [17]. Repression of p16 by promoter methylation is the most frequent alteration [20]. In addition, increased expression of Id1, an inhibitor of p16, is correlated with the HCC risk in cirrhotic patients as well as the expression of gankyrin, an inhibitor of the p53 and Rb checkpoints, is frequently increased in HCCs [21-22].

BRCA2

In addition to p53, another molecule involved in the DNA damage response is BRCA2. Loss of heterozygosity (LOH) of the BRCA2 locus has been documented in HCCs, providing genomic instability.

Betacatenin

Betacatenin overexpression and mutations have been related to early-stage HCCs and, in other studies, to HCC progression, and occur more frequently in HCV-related HCCs compared with HBV-related ones. However, it is also described a crucial role of HBx protein in betacatenin stabilization in hepatoma cells, demonstrating betacatenin role also in HBV-related HCCs [23]. Human HCCs characterized by high rates of genomic instability, and so with increased loss of heterozygosity (LOH), show very low levels of betacatenin mutations [24]. This highlights how betacatenin mutations are typical in HCCs with lower or absent levels of genomic instability.

MMP and RhoC

Expression of genes involved in regulation of extracellular matrix or cell motility as MMP14 and Rho C is increased in HCCs with the vascular invasion phenotype [13]. Matrix metalloproteinases (MMPs) are implicated in cancer invasion by degrading extracellular matrices. In HCC, expression of MMP14 mRNA is associated with poorer differentiation and poor outcome [25]. Rho is member of a family of small GTP-binding proteins involved in the cytoskeletal re-organization. Therefore Rho C overexpression is common in HCC and associated with increased tumor invasion and metastasis [26]. This observation is corroborated by the fact that Y-27632, a specific inhibitor of p160ROCK (p160 Rho-associated coiledcoil forming protein kinase) reduces the incidence of mice with metastatic nodules [27].

ErbB Receptor Family

The ErbB family of receptor tyrosine kinases consists of four members (ERBB1–ERBB4) that are involved in the development of different kind of human cancers. Overexpression of ERBB1 in 68% of HCC cases, ERBB2 (HER2) in 21%, ERBB3 in 84%, and ERBB4 in 61% have been described. ERBB1 and ERBB3 expression correlated with a more aggressive presentation that includes a high proliferation index and tumor size, de-differentiation and methastatic behaviour [28]. Many evidences for the ErbB receptor family involvement in hepatocarcinogenesis come from studies in mice. Interesting studies showed that mice transgenic for TGF, a ligand for ErbB receptors, develop HCCs [29]. Treatment with hepatocarcinogens accelerates HCC development in the TGFtransgenic strain; however, in TGF-deficient mice, smaller hepatic neoplasms are described [30]. The studies mentioned above underline the relevant role of the ERB pathways in HCC development and justify the interest to find therapies able to target this pathway.

MET and HGF

In advanced human HCC overexpression of the MET receptor has been described and several evidences show how important is this pathway in liver cancer. For example, transgenic mice for the c-MET ligand HGF, one of the most potent mitogens for hepatocytes, have been reported to develop HCCs by 1.5 years of age [31]. In another interesting study, the investigators demonstrated that liver expression of an activated MET transgene induced HCC development, and that the extinction of this gene expression resulted in apoptosis and decreased cell proliferation with consequent cancer regression [32].

Epigenetic Abnormalities

During the long preneoplastic stage and the early phases of HCC development, epigenetic abnormalities seem to have a predominant role, as demonstrated by several evidences. It is well known that the elevated expression of growth factors such as TGF-β or IGF-2 is responsible for accelerated hepatocyte proliferation in the earlier phase of hepatocarcinogenesis. Furthermore, it has been demonstrated that upregulation of these two genes is the result of the combined actions of cytokines and reflect the upregulation of several other genes by epigenetic mechanisms. The most emphasized epigenetic alteration in cancers is the aberrant hypermethylation of CpG islands. Several independent studies have revealed that DNA methylation in tumor suppressor genes can be found in non-cancerous liver tissues and this is an early event in cancer [33]. Also, in HCC several tumor suppressor genes are silenced by promoter methylations. APC, p16/INK4A, DLC1 are only few examples. In particular, p16 hypermethylation rate significantly increases from the transition of cirrhotic nodules (62.5%) to DNs (70.3%) or to HCCs with DNs (83.3%) [34]. Futher described hypermethylated genes are E-cadherin, RASSF1A, GTSP1, SOSC-1, SFRP1 and PTEN. In mammalian cells, DNA methylation is regulated by the activity of DNA methyltransferases (DNMTS). Aberrant expression of DNMTs can cause methylation errors or *de novo* methylations at normally unmethylated CpG sites. Several studies reported in human HCC an important overexpression of DNMT1, DNMT3A and DNMT3B. In a study by Choi et al, the authors showed that Dnmt1 and Dnmt3a could be involved in the early stage of hepatocarcinogenesis and that dysregulation of Dnmt3a may have a relevant role in cancer progression [35]. An upregulation of S-adenosylmethionine synthase and glycine N-methyltransferase, which augments the hepatocellular pool of methyl groups, has also been described in many HCCs. An interesting aspect is that different macroenvironment factors may influence epigenetic alterations. As regards the role of hepatitis B, DNA hypermethylation on GSTP1 and E-cadherin promoters are frequent in HCC-related to HBV infection [36]. In addition, HBV x protein (HBx) might regulate the expression of DNMTs [37]. Nutrition also plays an important role in epigenetic alterations. It is known that deficiency of the major dietary sources of methyl groups, including methionine, choline, folic acid and vitamin B-12 results in depletion of intracellular methyl group pools and may increase DNA hypomethylation [38]. Other influencing factors can be oxydative stress and flogosis. For example, oxidation of 5-methylcytosine to 5-hydroxymethylcytosine prevents DNMT1 methylation of cytosine in the opposite strand. In addition, inflammation-mediated damage products 5-chlorocytosine and 5-bromocytosine can mimic 5-methylcytosine. Dysregulation of DNA methylation caused by environmental factors may lead to global DNA hypomethylation and gene-specific DNA hypermethylation and this, in turn, may eventually result in chromosomal instability.

Several studies have tried to show the biological relevance of methylation of specific genes in order to propose therapeutic interventions. For example, in an interesting study, investigators showed that treatment of hepatoma cells with a demethylating agent increases p16 (INK4a) [39] and COX2 expression [40] with a consequent inhibition of cell proliferation. Further studies will be necessary to better understand the consequences of specific epigenetic gene silencing in cancer in order to propose new targeted drug therapies.

Signaling Pathways Involved in HCC Development

As a consequence of the genetic, epigenetic and chromosomal alterations described above several signaling pathways could be activated and dysregulated in HCC. Herein are reported some of the most studied signaling pathways.

1) The Wnt/β-catenin signaling pathway is a relevant signaling transduction pathway in the regulation of cell proliferation and motility and its activation is commonly detected in HCC. In the absence of Wnt signals, β-catenin is recruited to the degradation complex consisting of APC, Axin and glycogen synthase kinase (GSK)-3b. When bound to this complex, β-catenin is phosphorylated by GSK-3b and degradated through the ubiquitin–proteasome system. This continuous degradation contributes to maintain β-catenin at a low level steady state. When Wnt ligands bind to the transmembrane co-receptors frizzled and low-density lipoprotein receptor-related protein 5/6 (LRP5/6), Wnt/b-catenin signaling transduction is triggered. As a consequence, Dv1 is activated by phosphorylation and binds to GSK-3b, suppressing the kinase activity. Accumulation of the free, hypophosphorylated β-catenin in the cytoplasmic pool facilitates its nuclear translocation, where β-catenin forms a complex with transcription factors and upregulates the expression of several target genes such as c-Myc, cyclin D1, COX2, and MMP7. In human HCC, APC mutations are rarely detected and there is evidence that promoter methylation is implicated in APC inactivation [41]. Other described gene mutations are β-catenin (about 20-40% of HCCs, more frequently in HCV-related HCCs) and Axin1 (about 5-10%) [42-43]. As mentioned above, β-catenin is stabilized by HBx protein in HBV-related HCC. In addition, overexpression of Wnt ligand, Frizzled receptor, Dvl, PIN1 and sFRP1 has been reported in HCC. Instead, Dvl inhibitors, HDPR1 and Prickle-1 are frequently underexpressed [44-48].

2) Ras proteins, consisting of N-Ras, H-Ras and K-Ras are 21 kDa GTPases and are generally considered proto-oncogenes. Ras signaling is initiated when a ligand (e.g. EGF) binds to its membrane receptor and induces phosphorylation of tyrosine residues on its cytoplasmic domain, producing binding sites for proteins with SH2 domains such as GRB2. Ras protein, after conversion to its active GTP-bound form by SOS protein or other Ras guanine nucleotide exchange factors (RasGEF), activates the RAF/MEK/ERK pathway. Hyperphosphorylated ERK1/2 translocates into the nucleus and regulates the expression of target genes. Overexpression of Ras proteins and downregulation of several inhibitors of Ras/Raf/MEK/ERK pathways such as RKIP and Spred-1 have been detected in HCC and cirrhosis [49-51]. Activation of Ras signaling is usually associated with cellular transformation. However, a role in cell senescence and apoptosis can also been exerted by of the Ras signaling pathway likely trough RASSF1, which is frequently epigenetically silenced in HCC [52-53].

3) The TGF-β signaling pathway is believed to be an important mediator in cancer development from fibrosis. TGF-β1 is overexpressed in HCC, peri-neoplastic stroma [54], and cirrhosis and crucial in the induction of HSCs proliferation and activation with consequent collagen production [55]. Kluwe et al. showed that pan-JNK inhibitors prevent PDGF, TGF-β1 and angiotensin II-induced HSCs activation in mouse models, demonstrating the role of JNK as a mediator of TGF activity [56]. Another mediator of the TGF-β action in fibrogenesis is connective tissue growth factor (CCN2, also known as CTGF) [57]. TGF-β1 is a pleiotropic factor not only relevant in fibrogenesis. For example, TGF-β1 can act as a tumor suppressor in preneoplastic stage involving both hepatocytes and tumor microenvironment cellular components. The tumor suppressor activity of TGF-β1 includes anti-proliferative and proapoptotic effects mediated by the mobilization of cyclin-dependent kinase inhibitors, c-Myc suppression and down regulation of anti-apoptotic proteins [58]. The TGF-β1 activity may shift from tumor suppressor to oncogenic trough different mechanisms. It is noteworthy that HBx and HCV through JNK activation may shift the hepatocytic TGF-β signaling from a tumor-suppressive (pSmad3C) to an oncogenic pathway (pSmad3L) [59]. Another mechanism involved in this shift is the promoter methylation of tristetrapolin (TTP), a negative regulator of c-Myc at posttrascriptional level [60]. TGF-β1 can also modulate the oncogenic miRNA expression including miR-181b, -23a, -27a, and -24 to promote cell growth, survival and migration of cancer cells [61-62]. Furthermore, TGF-β1 is involved in several processes underlying cancer progression such as tumor cell migration, tumor–stromal crosstalk and angiogenesis, through the involvement of a number of growth factors including VEGF and CTGF (Figure 4) [63-64].

4) An activation of Akt signaling and reduced expression of phosphatase and tensin homolog (PTEN) (a Akt negative regulator) has been reported in 40%–60% of human HCCs, demonstrating the importance of this signaling pathway [65]. Akt pathway suppresses TGF-β-induced apoptosis and CCAAT/enhancer binding protein α growth-inhibitory activity, supporting cancer formation at the cirrhosis stage.

5) Lysophosphatidic acid (LPA) is a bioactive phospholipid with growth factor-like activity that sustains liver cancer formation. Several evidences support the role of LPA in cancer. For example, different cancer cell lines release into the culture medium significant amounts of lysophosphatidylcholine (LPC), a substrate for Autotaxin (ATX), the major LPA-producing enzyme [66]. Transcripts of ATX are elevated in HCC and there is a correlation between increased serum levels of LPA and α-fetoprotein

(AFP) [67]. LPA receptors (LPARs) are expressed differently in human HCC. One of these, LPAR6 is barely undetectable in normal hepatocytes, but it is significantly increased in HCC and documented to be involved in HCC tumorigenicity [68]. LPA is abundantly released from cancer cells as consequence of the enzymatic action of ATX and can act with an autocrine or paracrine mechanism stimulating cancer cell growth and the interaction of cancer cells with stromal cells (Figure 5). LPA influences and regulates cell migration by initiating reorganization of the actin cytoskeleton and it is also involved in the regulation of membrane ruffling (lamellipodia movement) and focal adhesion contacts. Because of its role in cell motitlity, LPA is considered an important factor in mediating HCC invasion.

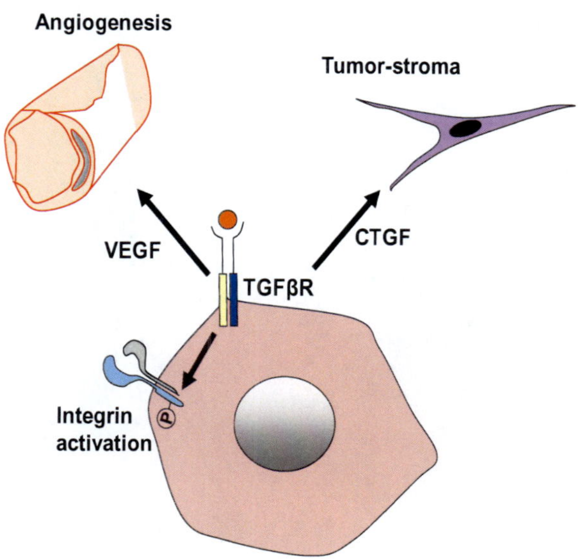

Figure 4. Transforming Growth Factor Beta1 (TGF-β1)-mediated pathways in HCC progression. TGFβ1 is involved in several biological pathways including fibrogenesis and cancer development and progression through the activation of VEGF, CTGF and integrin signaling which regulate angiogenesis and tumor-stroma crosstalk.

For example, treatment with LPA resulted in a dose-dependent increased in HuH7 cell growth and motility [69] and pharmacological inhibition of p38 MAPK signal pathway, a downstream mediator of LPA, reduced cell migration, invasion, and adhesion [70]. Several studies have demonstrated the implication of LPA in angiogenesis. LPA may induce VEGF expression in ovarian cancer cells through the activation of the hypoxia-inducible factor 1-

alpha (HIF-1A). In turn, VEGF promotes LPA production by inducing ATX expression [71]. Another interesting aspect to underline is the significant connection of LPA to cancer behavior. For example, elevated LPA serum levels are associated with larger and metastatic HCCs and shorter survival. LPA could also be important in the step-by step process from liver fibrosis to cancer since fibrosis is associated with increased ATX and LPA levels. Studies show that plasma LPA levels and serum ATX activity in mouse models were increased in carbon tetrachloride-induced liver fibrosis correlatively with fibrosis grade [72]. In addition, ATX serum levels correlate with liver cirrhosis severity (Child Pugh and Meld scores) [73]. Therefore, as supported by several evidences and considering the many biological activities of the ATX/LPA signaling axis, circulating LPA levels have been proposed as diagnostic and prognostic marker in patients with HCC.

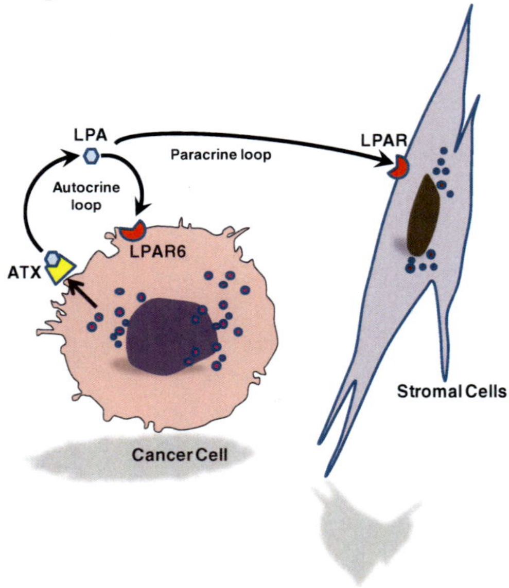

Figure 5. Involvement of lysophosphatidic acid (LPA) in HCC development. LPA is secreted from cancer cells as consequence of the enzymatic action of autotaxin (ATX) and acts in both autocrine and paracrine fashion stimulating the cancer cell growth and the interaction with cancer stromal cells.

6) Certain plasma membrane components can be organized in microdomains and regulate cell signaling pathways. Tetraspanins are transmembrane proteins defined by small and large extracellular loops, short N-terminal and C-terminal tails with four transmembrane domains that form complexes termed tetraspanin-enriched microdomains (TEMs) by

interacting with several proteins such as integrins, G proteins, proteases, immunoglobulins and cytosolic signal transduction molecules. Several tetraspanins including CD9, CD63, CD81, CD151 have been implicated in the regulation of cell proliferation, migration and cell fusion/exocytosis [74]. CD81 is a ubiquitously expressed tetraspanin protein. Interaction of CD81 with PI4KII suppresses HCC cell motility by promoting the formation of CD81-enriched vesicles that sequester actinin-4 with consequent remodelling of actin cytoskeleton [75]. CD81 induces reorganization of the plasma membrane and amplifyies the instability of pre-malignant hepatocytes. CD81 overexpression makes HCC cells unable to metastasize whereas CD81 decreased expression is associated with intrahepatic metastasis and poor differentiation. During hepatocytes-transformation, CD81 gene expression is progressively lost. Re-expression of CD81 in HCC cells preserves the capability to form the main tumor mass when injected intrahepatically into nude rats, but fails to produce tumors in distant parts of the liver (intrahepatic metastases) [75-76]. Another relevant feature of CD81 is the interaction with hepatitis C virus. Since CD81 binds to the E2 envelope glycoprotein of the HCV and functions as putative HCV-receptor, CD81 gene polymorphisms may correlate with certain clinical courses of HCV infection [77].

7) Proteolytic enzymes are involved in several processes dysregulated in cancer, such as cell detachment from the primary tumor, vessel wall crossing and extravasation into target organs that are the prerequisites of cancer invasion and metastasis. Expression and activity of several classes of proteolytic enzymes are modified in cancer including the recently discovered ADAMTS (A Disintegrin And Metalloproteinase with ThromboSpondin motifs). ADAMTS are metalloproteases synthesized as zymogens and secreted from cells after proteolytic processing at the N-terminal extremity. These enzymes are able to hydrolyze specific extracellular proteins. ADAMTS-1, -4 and -5 are able to cleave members of the hyalectan or lectican family of proteoglycans and are expressed at differential levels in hepatocellular carcinoma cell lines. Several activities have been attributed to ADAMTS. For example, ADAMTS-1 exerts pro and anti-angiogenic activities. ADAMTS-4 is involved in cancer progression and anti-angiogenic activities. Anti-angiogenic ADAMTS-5 protein is expressed at low levels by primary HCCs and this could allow tumoral angiogenesis. ADAMTS-1, ADAMTS-4 and ADAMTS-5 proteolytic activity is tightly regulated by the endogenous tissue inhibitor of metalloproteases 3 (TIMP3). The N-terminal domain of TIMPs provides its inhibitory action trough a non-covalent binary complex. Interaction of TIMP3 with ECM proteoglycans may enable TIMP3 to inhibit extracellular

ADAMTS. Under normal physiological conditions, TIMP3 regulates the proteolytic activity of ADAMTS, preventing their pathological effects. Dysregulated expression of TIMPs can occur at various stages of cancer progression and downregulation of TIMPs has been associated with increased tumor cell invasion [78].

8) Another class of molecules biologically relevant in liver cancer is the integrin family of extracellular matrix (ECM) receptors. Integrins are surface receptor proteins involved in modulation of adhesions between cells and between cells and ECM proteins. More than 20 integrin heterodimers are described derived from different splicing and combinations of alfa and beta subunits. Normal hepatocytes express only low levels of integrin α1β1, α5β1 and α9β1, however, in pathological conditions such as liver fibrosis or cancer, integrin α2β1, α3β1, α6β1 and α6β4 are found upregulated. Several studies have demonstrated that HCC patients characterized by multiple nodules, vascular invasion and the absence of encapsulation exhibit increased α6β1 expression. This increased expression in HCC cells seems to be necessary for FAK/MAP kinase-dependent migration [79-80]. In addition to the α6β1 activity in cell adesion and migration, another crucial role of this integrin in carcinogenesis consists in providing a ligand-independent growth advantage or a specific growth pathway by regulating cellular architecture. Among other well-studied integrins involved in HCC progression, α3β1 integrin is overexpressed and associated with increased invasiveness of HCC cells. α3β1 integrin is also involved in the molecular network that regulates the interactions between HCC cells and microenvironment. On the contrary, β3 integrin, which regulates cell growth inibition and apoptosis, is underexpressed in HCC [81].

References

[1] Marchio A, Meddeb M, Pineau P, Danglot G, Tiollais P, Bernheim A, Dejean A. 1997. "Recurrent chromosomal abnormalities in hepatocellular carcinoma detected by comparative genomic hybridization." *Genes Chromosomes Cancer* 18:59-65.

[2] Yu CT, Hsu JM, Lee YC, Tsou AP, Chou CK, Huang CY. 2005. "Phosphorylation and stabilization of HURP by Aurora-A: implication of HURP as a transforming target of Aurora-A." *Mol Cell Biol* 25:5789-800.

[3] Saeki A, Tamura S, Ito N, Kiso S, Matsuda Y, Yabuuchi I, Kawata S, Matsuzawa Y. 2002. “Frequent impairment of the spindle assembly checkpoint in hepatocellular carcinoma.” *Cancer* 94:2047-54.

[4] Bruix J, Boix L, Sala M, Llovet JM. 2004. “Focus on hepatocellular carcinoma.” *Cancer Cell* 5:215-9.

[5] Yamada T, De Souza AT, Finkelstein S, Jirtle RL. 1997. “Loss of the gene encoding mannose 6-phosphate/insulin-like growth factor II receptor is an early event in liver carcinogenesis.” *Proc Natl Acad Sci U S A* 94:10351-5.

[6] Oh BK, Kim YJ, Park C, Park YN. 2005. “Up-regulation of telomere-binding proteins, TRF1, TRF2, and TIN2 is related to telomere shortening during human multistep hepatocarcinogenesis.” *Am J Pathol* 166:73-80.

[7] Farazi PA, Glickman J, Jiang S, Yu A, Rudolph KL, DePinho RA. 2003. “Differential impact of telomere dysfunction on initiation and progression of hepatocellular carcinoma.” Cancer Res 63:5021-7.

[8] Farazi PA, DePinho RA. 2006. “Hepatocellular carcinoma pathogenesis: from genes to environment.” *Nat Rev Cancer* 6:674-87.

[9] Parrinello S, Coppe JP, Krtolica A, Campisi J. 2005. “Stromal-epithelial interactions in aging and cancer: senescent fibroblasts alter epithelial cell differentiation.” *J Cell Sci* 118:485-96.

[10] Choudhury AR, Ju Z, Djojosubroto MW, Schienke A, Lechel A, Schaetzlein S, Jiang H, Stepczynska A, Wang C, Buer J, Lee HW, von Zglinicki T, Ganser A, Schirmacher P, Nakauchi H, Rudolph KL. 2007. “Cdkn1a deletion improves stem cell function and lifespan of mice with dysfunctional telomeres without accelerating cancer formation.” *Nat Genet* 39:99-105.

[11] Wagayama H, Shiraki K, Yamanaka T, Sugimoto K, Ito T, Fujikawa K, Takase K, Nakano T. 2001. “p21WAF1/CTP1 expression and hepatitis virus type.” *Dig Dis Sci* 46:2074-9.

[12] Laurent-Puig P, Legoix P, Bluteau O, Belghiti J, Franco D, Binot F, Monges G, Thomas G, Bioulac-Sage P, Zucman-Rossi J. 2001. “Genetic alterations associated with hepatocellular carcinomas define distinct pathways of hepatocarcinogenesis.” *Gastroenterology* 120:1763-73.

[13] Okabe H, Satoh S, Kato T, Kitahara O, Yanagawa R, Yamaoka Y, Tsunoda T, Furukawa Y, Nakamura Y. 2001. “Genome-wide analysis of gene expression in human hepatocellular carcinomas using cDNA microarray: identification of genes involved in viral carcinogenesis and tumor progression.” *Cancer Res* 61:2129-37.

[14] Wong CM, Ng IO. 2008. "Molecular pathogenesis of hepatocellular carcinoma." *Liver Int* 28:160-74.

[15] Kim CM, Koike K, Saito I, Miyamura T, Jay G. 1991. "HBx gene of hepatitis B virus induces liver cancer in transgenic mice." *Nature* 351:317-20.

[16] El-Serag HB, Rudolph KL. 2007. "Hepatocellular Carcinoma: Epidemiology and Molecular Carcinogenesis." *Gastroenterology* 132: 2557-76.

[17] Plentz RR, Park YN, Lechel A, Kim H, Nellessen F, Langkopf BH, Wilkens L, Destro A, Fiamengo B, Manns MP, Roncalli M, Rudolph KL. 2007. "Telomere shortening and inactivation of cell cycle checkpoints characterize human hepatocarcinogenesis." *Hepatology* 45: 968-76.

[18] Ghebranious N, Sell S. 1998. "The mouse equivalent of the human p53ser249 mutation p53ser246 enhances aflatoxin hepatocarcinogenesis in hepatitis B surface antigen transgenic and p53 heterozygous null mice."*Hepatology* 27:967-73.

[19] Ghebranious N, Sell S. 1998. "Hepatitis B injury, male gender, aflatoxin, and p53 expression each contribute to hepatocarcinogenesis in transgenic mice." *Hepatology* 27:383-91.

[20] Azechi H, Nishida N, Fukuda Y, Nishimura T, Minata M, Katsuma H, Kuno M, Ito T, Komeda T, Kita R,Takahashi R, Nakao K. 2001. "Disruption of the p16/cyclin D1/retinoblastoma protein pathway in the majority of human hepatocellular carcinomas." *Oncology* 60: 346-54.

[21] Matsuda Y, Yamagiwa S, Takamura M, Honda Y, Ishimoto Y, Ichida T, Aoyagi Y. 2005. "Overexpressed Id-1 is associated with a high risk of hepatocellular carcinoma development in patients with cirrhosis without transcriptional repression of p16." *Cancer* 104:1037-44.

[22] Higashitsuji H, Itoh K, Nagao T, Dawson S, Nonoguchi K, Kido T, Mayer RJ, Arii S, Fujita J. 2000."Reduced stability of retinoblastoma protein by gankyrin, an oncogenic ankyrin-repeat protein overexpressed in hepatomas." *Nat Med* 6: 96-9.

[23] Cha MY, Kim CM, Park YM, Ryu WS. 2004. "Hepatitis B virus X protein is essential for the activation of Wnt/beta-catenin signaling in hepatoma cells." *Hepatology* 39:1683-93.

[24] Gross-Goupil M, Riou P, Emile JF, Saffroy R, Azoulay D, Lacherade I, Receveur A, Piatier-Tonneau D, Castaing D, Debuire B, Lemoine A. 2003. "Analysis of chromosomal instability in pulmonary or liver

metastases and matched primary hepatocellular carcinoma after orthotopic liver transplantation." *Int J Cancer* 104:745-51.

[25] Määttä M, Soini Y, Liakka A, Autio-Harmainen H. 2000. "Differential expression of matrix metalloproteinase (MMP)-2, MMP -9, and membrane type 1-MMP in hepatocellular and pancreatic adenocarcinoma: implications for tumor progression and clinical prognosis." *Clin Cancer Res* 6:2726-34.

[26] Wang W, Yang LY, Huang GW, Lu WQ, Yang ZL, Yang JQ, Liu HL. 2004. "Genomic analysis reveals RhoC as a potential marker in hepatocellular carcinoma with poor prognosis." *Br J Cancer* 90:2349-55.

[27] Takamura M, Sakamoto M, Genda T, Ichida T, Asakura H, Hirohashi S. 2001. "Inhibition of intrahepatic metastasis of human hepatocellular carcinoma by Rho-associated protein kinase inhibitor Y-27632." *Hepatology.* 33:577-81.

[28] Ito Y, Takeda T, Sakon M, Tsujimoto M, Higashiyama S, Noda K, Miyoshi E, Monden M, Matsuura N. 2001. "Expression and clinical significance of erb-B receptor family in hepatocellular carcinoma." *Br J Cancer* 84:1377-83.

[29] Jhappan C, Stahle C, Harkins RN, Fausto N, Smith GH, Merlino GT. 1990. "TGF alpha overexpression in transgenic mice induces liver neoplasia and abnormal development of the mammary gland and pancreas." *Cell* 61:1137-46.

[30] Russell WE, Kaufmann WK, Sitaric S, Luetteke NC, Lee DC. 1996. "Liver regeneration and hepatocarcinogenesis in transforming growth factor-alpha-targeted mice." *Mol Carcinog* 15:183-9.

[31] Sakata H, Takayama H, Sharp R, Rubin JS, Merlino G, LaRochelle WJ. 1996. "Hepatocyte growth factor/scatter factor overexpression induces growth, abnormal development, and tumor formation in transgenic mouse livers." *Cell Growth Differ* 7:1513-23.

[32] Wang R, Ferrell LD, Faouzi S, Maher JJ, Bishop JM. 2001. "Activation of the Met receptor by cell attachment induces and sustains hepatocellular carcinomas in transgenic mice." *J Cell Biol* 153:1023-34.

[33] Kondo Y, Shen L, Suzuki S, Kurokawa T, Masuko K, Tanaka Y, Kato H, Mizuno Y, Yokoe M, Sugauchi F, Hirashima N, Orito E, Osada H, Ueda R, Guo Y, Chen X, Issa JP, Sekido Y. 2007. "Alterations of DNA methylation and histone modifications contribute to gene silencing in hepatocellular carcinomas." *Hepatol Res* 37:974-83.

[34] Liew CT, Li HM, Lo KW, Leow CK, Chan JY, Hin LY, Lau WY, Lai PB, Lim BK, Huang J, Leung WT, Wu S, Lee JC. 1999. "High

frequency of p16INK4A gene alterations in hepatocellular carcinoma." *Oncogene* 18:789-95.

[35] Choi MS, Shim YH, Hwa JY, Lee SK, Ro JY, Kim JS, Yu E. 2003. "Expression of DNA methyltransferases in multistep hepatocarcinogenesis." *Hum Pathol* 34:11-7.

[36] Su PF, Lee TC, Lin PJ, Lee PH, Jeng YM, Chen CH, Liang JD, Chiou LL, Huang GT, Lee HS. 2007. "Differential DNA methylation associated with hepatitis B virus infection in hepatocellular carcinoma." *Int J Cancer* 121:1257-64.

[37] Park IY, Sohn BH, Yu E, Suh DJ, Chung YH, Lee JH, Surzycki SJ, Lee YI. 2007. "Aberrant epigenetic modifications in hepatocarcinogenesis induced by hepatitis B virus X protein." *Gastroenterology* 132:1476-94.

[38] Pogribny IP, Ross SA, Wise C, Pogribna M, Jones EA, Tryndyak VP, James SJ, Dragan YP, Poirier LA. 2006. "Irreversible global DNA hypomethylation as a key step in hepatocarcinogenesis induced by dietary methyl deficiency." *Mutat Res* 593:80-7.

[39] Maeta Y, Shiota G, Okano J, Murawaki Y. 2005. "Effect of promoter methylation of the p16 gene on phosphorylation of retinoblastoma gene product and growth of hepatocellular carcinoma cells." *Tumour Biol* 26:300-5.

[40] Murata H, Tsuji S, Tsujii M, Sakaguchi Y, Fu HY, Kawano S, Hori M. 2004. "Promoter hypermethylation silences cyclooxygenase-2 (Cox-2) and regulates growth of human hepatocellular carcinoma cells." *Lab Invest* 84:1050-9.

[41] Yang B, Guo M, Herman JG, Clark DP. 2003. "Aberrant promoter methylation profiles of tumor suppressor genes in hepatocellular carcinoma." *Am J Pathol* 163:1101-7.

[42] Huang H, Fujii H, Sankila A, Mahler-Araujo BM, Matsuda M, Cathomas G, Ohgaki H. 1999. "Beta-catenin mutations are frequent in human hepatocellular carcinomas associated with hepatitis C virus infection." *Am J Pathol* 155:1795-801.

[43] Taniguchi K, Roberts LR, Aderca IN, Dong X, Qian C, Murphy LM, Nagorney DM, Burgart LJ, Roche PC, Smith DI, Ross JA, Liu W. 2002. "Mutational spectrum of beta-catenin, AXIN1, and AXIN2 in hepatocellular carcinomas and hepatoblastomas." *Oncogene* 21:4863-71.

[44] Lee TH, Tai DI, Cheng CJ, Sun CS, Lin CY, Sheu MJ, Lee WP, Peng CY, Wang AH, Tsai SL. 2006. "Enhanced nuclear factorkappa B-associated Wnt-1 expression in hepatitis B- and C related

hepatocarcinogenesis: identification by functional proteomics." *J Biomed Sci* 13:27-39.
[45] Merle P, Kim M, Herrmann M, Gupte A, Lefrançois L, Califano S, Trépo C, Tanaka S, Vitvitski L, de la Monte S, Wands JR. 2005. "Oncogenic role of the frizzled-7/beta-catenin pathway in hepatocellular carcinoma." *J Hepatol* 43:854-62.
[46] Chan DW, Chan CY, Yam JW, Ching YP, Ng IO. 2006. "Prickle-1 negatively regulates Wnt/beta-catenin pathway by promoting Dishevelled ubiquitination /degradation in liver cancer." *Gastroenterology* 131:1218-27.
[47] Pang R, Yuen J, Yuen MF, Lai CL, Lee TK, Man K, Poon RT, Fan ST, Wong CM, Ng IO, Kwong YL, Tse E. 2004. "PIN1 overexpression and beta catenin gene mutations are distinct oncogenic events in human hepatocellular carcinoma." *Oncogene* 23:4182-6.
[48] Yau TO, Chan CY, Chan KL, Lee MF, Wong CM, Fan ST, Ng IO. 2005. "HDPR1, a novel inhibitor of the WNT/beta-catenin signaling, is frequently downregulated in hepatocellular carcinoma: involvement of methylation mediated gene silencing." *Oncogene* 24:1607-14.
[49] Nonomura A, Ohta G, Hayashi M, Izumi R, Watanabe K, Takayanagi N, Mizukami Y, Matsubara F. 1987 "Immunohistochemical detection of ras oncogene p21 product in liver cirrhosis and hepatocellular carcinoma." *Am J Gastroenterol* 82:512-8.
[50] Schuierer MM, Bataille F, Weiss TS, Hellerbrand C, Bosserhoff AK. 2006. "Raf kinase inhibitor protein is downregulated in hepatocellular carcinoma." *Oncol Rep* 16:451-6.
[51] Yoshida T, Hisamoto T, Akiba J, Koga H, Nakamura K, Tokunaga Y, Hanada S, Kumemura H, Maeyama M, Harada M, Ogata H, Yano H, Kojiro M, Ueno T,Yoshimura A, Sata M. 2006. "Spreds, inhibitors of the Ras/ERK signal transduction, are dysregulated in human hepatocellular carcinoma and linked to the malignant phenotype of tumors." *Oncogene* 25:6056-66.
[52] Serrano M, Lin AW, McCurrach ME, Beach D, Lowe SW. 1997. "Oncogenic ras provokes premature cell senescence associated with accumulation of p53 and p16INK4a." *Cell* 88:593-602.
[53] Downward J. 1998. "Ras signalling and apoptosis." *Curr Opin Genet Dev* 8: 49-54.
[54] Bedossa P, Peltier E, Terris B, Franco D, Poynard T. 1995. "Transforming growth factor-beta 1 (TGF-beta 1) and TGF-beta 1

receptors in normal, cirrhotic, and neoplastic human livers." *Hepatology* 21:760–6.

[55] Eghbali-Fatourechi G, Sieck GC, Prakash YS, Maercklein P, Gores GJ, Fitzpatrick LA. 1996. "Type I procollagen production and cell proliferation is mediated by transforming growth factor-beta in a model of hepatic fibrosis." *Endocrinology* 137:1894-903.

[56] Kluwe J, Pradere JP, Gwak GY, Mencin A, De Minicis S, Osterreicher CH, Colmenero J, Bataller R, and Schwabe RF. 2010. "Modulation of hepatic fibrosis by c-Jun-N-terminal kinase inhibition." *Gastroenterology* 138:347-59. Accessed September 24, 2009. doi: 10.1053/j.gastro.2009.09.015.

[57] Gao R, Brigstock DR. 2004. "Connective tissue growth factor (CCN2) induces adhesion of rat activated hepatic stellate cells by binding of its C-terminal domain to integrin alpha(v)beta(3) and heparan sulfate proteoglycan." *J Biol Chem* 279:8848-55.

[58] Massagué J. 2008. "TGFbeta in Cancer." *Cell* 134:215-30. doi: 10.1016/j.cell.2008.07.001.

[59] Murata M, Matsuzaki K, Yoshida K, Sekimoto G, Tahashi Y, Mori S, Uemura Y, Sakaida N, Fujisawa J, Seki T, Kobayashi K, Yokote K, Koike K, Okazaki K. 2009. "Hepatitis B virus X protein shifts human hepatic transforming growth factor (TGF)beta signaling from tumorsuppression to oncogenesis in early chronic hepatitis B." *Hepatology* 49:1203-17. doi: 10.1002/hep.22765.

[60] Sohn BH, Park IY, Lee JJ, Yang SJ, Jang YJ, Park KC, Kim DJ, Lee DC, Sohn HA, Kim TW, Yoo HS, Choi JY, Bae YS, and Yeom YI. 2010. "Functional switching of TGF-beta1 signaling in liver cancer via epigenetic modulation of a single CpG site in TTP promoter." *Gastroenterology* 138:1898-908. Accessed December 29, 2009. doi: 10.1053/j.gastro.2009.12.044.

[61] Wang B, Hsu SH, Majumder S, Kutay H, Huang W, Jacob ST, Ghoshal K. 2010. "TGFbeta-mediated upregulation of hepatic miR-181b promotes hepato-carcinogenesis by targeting TIMP3." *Oncogene* 29:1787-97. Accessed December 21, 2009. doi: 10.1038/onc.2009.468.

[62] Huang S, He X, Ding J, Liang L, Zhao Y, Zhang Z, Yao X, Pan Z, Zhang P, Li J, Wan D, and Gu J. 2008. "Upregulation of miR-23a approximately 27a approximately 24 decreases transforming growth factor-beta-induced tumor-suppressive activities in human hepatocellular carcinoma cells." *Int J Cancer* 123:972-8. doi: 10.1002/ijc.23580.

[63] Mazzocca A, Fransvea E, Lavezzari G, Antonaci S, and Giannelli G. 2009. "Inhibition of transforming growth factor beta receptor I kinase blocks hepatocellular carcinoma growth through neo-angiogenesis regulation." *Hepatology* 50:1140-51. doi: 10.1002/hep.23118.

[64] Mazzocca A, Fransvea E, Dituri F, Lupo L, Antonaci S, and Giannelli G. 2010. "Down-regulation of connective tissue growth factor by inhibition of transforming growth factor beta blocks the tumor-stroma cross-talk and tumor progression in hepatocellular carcinoma." *Hepatology* 51:523-34. doi: 10.1002/hep.23285.

[65] Hu TH, Huang CC, Lin PR, Chang HW, Ger LP, Lin YW, Changchien CS, Lee CM, Tai MH. 2003. "Expression and prognostic role of tumor suppressor gene PTEN/MMAC1/TEP1 in hepatocellular carcinoma." *Cancer* 97:1929-40.

[66] Umezu-Goto M, Kishi Y, Taira A, Hama K, Dohmae N, Takio K, Yamori T, Mills GB, Inoue K, Aoki J,Arai H. 2002. "Autotaxin has lysophospholipase D activity leading to tumor cell growth and motility by lysophosphatidic acid production." *J Cell Biol* 158:227-33.

[67] Patterson AD, Maurhofer O, Beyoglu D, Lanz C, Krausz KW, Pabst T, Gonzalez FJ, Dufour JF, Idle JR. 2011. "Aberrant lipid metabolism in hepatocellular carcinoma revealed by plasma metabolomics and lipid profiling." *Cancer Res* 71:6590-600.

[68] Mazzocca A, Dituri F, De Santis F, Filannino A, Lopane C, Betz RC, Li YY, Mukaida N, Winter P, Tortorella C, Giannelli G, Sabbà C. 2015. "Lysophosphatidic acid receptor LPAR6 supports the tumorigenicity of hepatocellular Carcinoma." *Cancer Res* 75:532-43.

[69] Sokolov E, Eheim AL, Ahrens WA, Walling TL, Swet JH, McMillan MT, Simo KA, Thompson KJ, Sindram D, and McKillop IH. 2013. "Lysophosphatidic acid receptor expression and function in human hepatocellular carcinoma." *J Surg Res* 180:104-13. Accessed November 15, 2012. doi: 10.1016/j.jss.2012.10.054.

[70] Zhu B, Shi S, Ma YG, Fan F, Yao ZZ. 2012. "Lysophosphatidic acid enhances human hepatocellular carcinoma cell migration, invasion and adhesion through P38 MAPK pathway." *Hepatogastroenterology* 59:785-9.

[71] Ptaszynska MM, Pendrak ML, Stracke ML, Roberts DD. 2010. "Autotaxin signaling via lysophosphatidic acid receptors contributes to vascular endothelial growth factor-induced endothelial cell migration." *Mol Cancer Res* 8:309-21.

[72] Watanabe N, Ikeda H, Nakamura K, Ohkawa R, Kume Y, Tomiya T, Tejima K, Nishikawa T, Arai M, Yanase M, Aoki J, Arai H, Omata M, Fujiwara K, Yatomi Y. 2007. "Plasma lysophosphatidic acid level and serum autotaxin activity are increased in liver injury in rats in relation to its severity." *Life Sci* 81: 1009-15.

[73] Pleli T, Martin D, Kronenberger B, Brunner F, Köberle V, Grammatikos G, Farnik H, Martinez Y, Finkelmeier F, Labocha S, Ferreirós N, Zeuzem S, Piiper A, and Waidmann O. 2014. "Serum autotaxin is a parameter for the severity of liver cirrhosis and overall survival in patients with liver cirrhosis: a prospective cohort study." *PLoS One* 9: e103532. doi: 10.1371/journal.pone.0103532.

[74] Mazzocca A, Carloni V, Sciammetta S, Cordella C, Pantaleo P, Caldini A, Gentilini P, Pinzani M. 2002. "Expression of transmembrane 4 superfamily (TM4SF) proteins and their role in hepatic stellate cell motility and wound healing migration." *J Hepatol* 37:322-30.

[75] Mazzocca A, Liotta F, Carloni V. 2008. "Tetraspanin CD81-regulated cell motility plays a critical role in intrahepatic metastasis of hepatocellular carcinoma." *Gastroenterology* 135:244-256.

[76] Inoue G, Horiike N, Onji M. 2001. "The CD81 expression in liver in hepatocellular carcinoma." *Int J Mol Med* 7:67-71.

[77] Itakura J, Nagayama K, Enomoto N, Sakamoto N, Tazawa J, Izumi N, Marumo F, Sato C. 2001. "CD81 nucleotide mutation in hepatocellular carcinoma and lack of CD81 polymorphism in patients at stages of hepatitis C virus infection." *J Med Virol* 63:22-8.

[78] Turner SL, Mangnall D, Bird NC, Bunning RA, Blair-Zajdel ME. 2012. "Expression of ADAMTS-1, ADAMTS-4, ADAMTS-5 and TIMP3 by hepatocellular carcinoma cell lines." *Int J Oncol* 41:1043-9.

[79] Nejjari M, Hafdi Z, Dumortier J, Bringuier AF, Feldmann G, Scoazec JY. 1999. "alpha6beta1 integrin expression in hepatocarcinoma cells: regulation and role in cell adhesion and migration." *Int J Cancer* 83:518-25.

[80] Carloni V, Mazzocca A, Pantaleo P, Cordella C, Laffi G, Gentilini P. 2001. "The integrin, alpha6beta1, is necessary for the matrix-dependent activation of FAK and MAP kinase and the migration of human hepatocarcinoma cells." *Hepatology* 34:42-9.

[81] Wu Y, Zuo J, Ji G, Saiyin H, Liu X, Yin F, Cao N, Wen Y, Li JJ, and Yu L. 2009. "Proapoptotic function of integrin beta (3) in human hepatocellular carcinoma cells." *Clin Cancer Res* 15:60-9. doi: 10.1158/1078-0432.

Chapter 4

Pathobiology of HCC: The Role of Microenvironment

For several decades, it has been thought that tumors develop because of growth pathway genes mutations with consequent alteration of the balance between oncogenes and oncosuppressor genes. It has now become clear that the activity of genes is often affected by epigenetic mechanisms and that environmental factors influence gene expression. Another breakthrough in the knowledge and comprehension of cancer formation and progression has come from studies that have underlined the role of the tissue microenvironment and its interaction with cancer cells. The tissue microenvironment includes different cell types such as hepatic stellate cells (HSCs), Kupffer cells, macrophages, endothelial cells and different protein components including extracellular matrix (ECM) proteins (laminins, collagens, fibronectin, vitronectin, fibrinogen), matrix metalloproteases (MMPs), serin proteases, growth factors as transforming growth factor-1 (TGF-β1) and hepatocyte growth factor (HGF).

The ECM environment is an important determinant of tumor cell behavior. There is evidence suggesting that HCC behavior can be predicted from knowledge of the pattern of genetic changes (molecular signatures) present in the nontumorous part of the liver. Using microarray techniques and proteomics, several investigators are studying the ''fingerprint'' of HCC compared to the peritumoral tissues, however, the interpretation of these results is yet unclear. The ability of a tumor to invade and metastasize is dependent on its ability to actively degrade ECM and by elaborating ECM degrading enzymes including MMPs. A MMP family member MT1-MMP may be the most important independent determinant of tumor invasion and has been proposed as a key gene of invasive HCC [1].

HSCs represent the main source of ECM production and can be recruited by tumor cells to produce the matrix degrading enzymes required for invasion in the context of a continuous balance between ECM production and degradation. After activation, HSCs express and secrete higher levels of collagens, above all fibrillar collagen type I, II and III, forming a contractile apparatus. The result is the aquisition of the ability to infiltrate HCC stroma and to localize around tumor sinusoids. This underlines that HSCs are not only a key cellular component in fibrosis, but also in HCC development and progression. Several authors observed that coculturing hepatocytes and the LX2 spontaneous immortalized human HSC cell line result in the induction of an inflammatory microenvironment and HCC proliferation and migration through a bidirectional crosstalk [2]. Another interesting evidence was that, in mice, subcutaneous coimplantation of human HSCs and HCC cells induced tumor development and invasiveness and inhibited necrosis [3].

Of similar importance for cancer development and progression is the paracrine crosstalk between cancer cells and carcinoma associated-fibroblasts (CAFs) [4] (Figure 6). At the interface between HCC and surrounding liver a wide range of patterns are seen. One of these patterns is known as encapsulation and is characterized by discrete layers of connective tissue and stromal cells. The capsule of HCC consists mostly of dense fibrillar collagen, with stable collagen I on its internal aspect adjacent to tumor, and a higher proportion of collagen III on the external one. However, encapsulation is not a simple "on or off" state and few tumors have a completely intact capsule. Several authors have demonstrated that encapsulation impacts on cancer behavior. Indeed, an association between tumor encapsulation and reduced cancer recurrence has been described [5]. The completeness of the capsule is probably more important than its thickness [6]. Myofibroblasts (MFBs) have been proposed as the principal source of collagen within tumor and the capsule and are present in high concentrations at the tumor-host interface. The density of MFBs decreases with increasing distance from the host-tumor interface. One probable explanation for this would be a diffusible factor secreted by tumor cells, promoting activation of resting HSCs, recruitment by chemotaxis of MFBs, or proliferation of MFBs already present. A relevant observation is that fibrogenic response in the surrounding parenchyma corresponds closely with the extent of collagen deposition within the tumor. Tumors with the greatest fibrogenic response in the surrounding tissue show enhanced cellular and vascular invasion and are usually surrounded by an incomplete peritumoral capsule. Higher levels of collagen I mRNA expression within tumor are positively associated with invasion, and less likely with a peritumoral capsule. However, the presence of a capsule reflects reduced invasiveness of the tumor [5]. In addition to ECM components, many evidences show the existence of tumor cell derived secreted extracellular membrane vesicles, also called exosomes or oncosomes, as carriers containing signaling proteins and genetic material, with different biological effects and potential influences in HCC initiation and progression. The matricellular proteins and ECM-associated proteins secreted by tumor or adjacent stromal cells have been widely described. As mentioned above, during the step-by-step process of hepatocarcinogenesis form chronic liver disease, changes in ECM proteins are determinant to the creation of a specific microenvironment, which could be considered as a network between tumor and stromal cells mediated by paracrine- and endocrine-secretion of growth factors, exosomes, or matricellular proteins, crucial in cancer development. The relationship between HCC and host stroma is an important determinant of the tumor growth pattern. This continuous crosstalk between HCC cells and the surrounding ECM proteins is mediated by integrins, metalloproteases, growth factors and cytokines. Platelet derived growth factor (PDGF), the most potent proliferative and chemotactic cytokine for HSCs or MFBs is also involved in mediating the host-tumor interactions. MFBs express both PDGF-BB and its receptor, thus allowing an autocrine loop. Connective tissue growth factor (CTGF) is a relevant mediator among the tumor-secreted factors involved in the crosstalk between cancer and stromal cells, as reported in a study where down-regulation of CTGF consequent to inhibition of TGF-β1 restrained the tumor-stroma crosstalk and HCC progression [7]. Considering that CTGF is a mediator of the TGF signaling pathway, this observation explains the role of TGF-β1 in this context. It has been reported that proteolytic cleavage by MMP-9 or MMP-2 activates latent TGF-β in tumor microenvironment and that this activation promotes tumor invasion and angiogenesis [8]. However, the proteolityc source of TGF-β in HCC is still uncharacterized. Probably, HCC cells or other surrounding cells such as myoepithelial or inflammatory cells are involved.

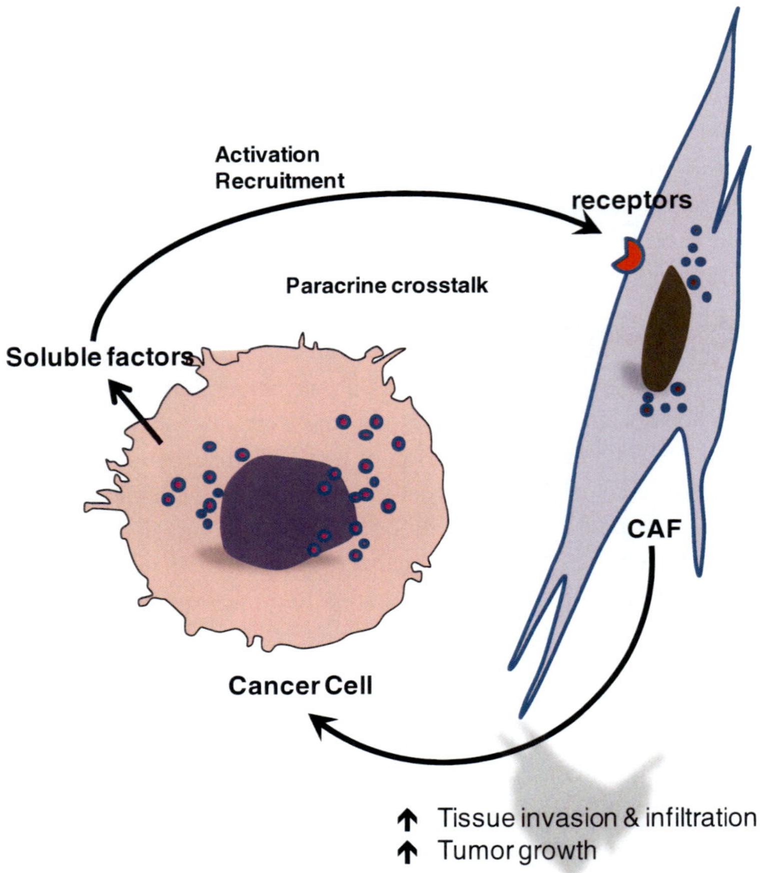

Figure 6. The tumor-stromal paracrine crosstalk pathways. The relation between cancer and stromal cells (carcinoma associated-fibroblasts/CAFs) is determinant for cancer development and progression. In this reciprocal crosstalk several soluble factors have a crucial role.

Liver Regeneration, Fibrosis and Inflammation

In animal models, liver regeneration after partial hepatectomy is arrested precisely when the hepatic structure is restored. By contrast, the continuous remodeling during liver cirrhosis creates an altered hepatic structure and eventually a growth-stimulatory microenvironment that accelerates cancer formation. Fibrogenesis, a process underlying tissue repair, is a dynamic mechanism characterized by synthesis of ECM proteins. When the noxious stimulus is timely arrested, the mechanism of tissue repair including tissue remodeling and epithelial regeneration leads to *restitutio ad integrum* of the liver parenchyma. In such conditions, fibrogenesis occurs but fibrosis, defined as the detectable deposit of ECM, is not usually observed. Instead, in the case of persistence of the noxious agent and prolonged liver injury, liver fibrosis occurs and represents the hallmark of chronic liver disease.

Liver fibrosis affects the portal space or the central vein. The preferential site for fibrosis to initiate largely depends on etiology (e.g. central fibrosis for vascular or alcoholic fibrosis and portal fibrosis for viral infections and autoimmune or biliary diseases). To this end, the activation of resident fibroblasts located within the central vein wall or portal tracts is determinant. The expansion of activated hepatic stellate cells (HSCs) and the fibrous tissue around the portal tract or central vein leads to the development of fibrous connections (bridging fibrosis) between vascular structures. This leads to the development of angiogenesis and at late stage of liver cirrhosis. ECM in the liver is not only a scaffold for liver architecture, but also a continuous network between cells that allows the continuous exchange of signals. These signals are favored by the storage within the ECM of numerous growth factors, hormones, enzymes, and cytokines in their inactive forms in a way that, after activation, they influence the microenvironment. One of the hallmarks of cirrhosis is the transactivation of HSCs into myofibroblasts, which produce and release ECM proteins, cytokines, growth factors, MMPs and oxidative stress-related factors. HSCs, also known as Ito cells, are pericytes-like cells located in the perisinusoidal space (space of Disse) representing a small percentage in normal liver (less than 10% of total resident liver cells). Quiescent HSCs are involved in metabolism and storage of retinoids, synthesis of growth factors and regulation of the sinusoidal blood flow. By contrast, activated HSCs transdifferentiate into myofibroblasts and express α-smooth muscle actin (α-SMA), the main histological hallmark of these cells. Activation of HSCs is also relevant in cancer development. Several data indicate that proliferation of hepatocytes is stimulated by activated HSCs secreted factors including insulin-like growth factor 1 (IGF-1), transforming growth factor alpha (TGF-α), hepatocyte growth factor (HGF) and inflammatory cytokines.

The mechanism of HSC activation has been divided into two steps: initiation and perpetuation. The early step is associated with rapid changes in gene expression making cells reactive to cytokines and growth factors. Oxidative stress and lipid peroxidation are the most important initiating factor in HSCs activation [9]. Reactive oxygen species (ROS) are generated by activated Kupffer cells, polymorphonucleates and damaged hepatocytes. After polyunsatured fatty acid degradation of the cell membrane, ROS lead to the production of different aldehydic end products. The aldehydic end product malondialdehyde and 4-hydroxy-2, 3-nonenal have been identified in different chronic liver diseases [10] and could be involved in several processes such as production of protein and DNA adducts, protein-polymerization and enzyme inactivation. A spliced variant of cellular fibronectin (EIIIA) produced by altered endothelial cells is another factor involved in the initiation phase [11]. Kupffer cells and endotelial cells are key cells involved in HSC activation. Regulation of several transcription genes could have a crucial role during early HSC activation and several transcription factors have been proposed including Sp1, c-myb, nuclear factor κB (NF-κB), STAT-1, and Zf9. The activated phenotype of HSCs is maintained and amplified by the perpetuation of mechanisms involving autocrine and paracrine stimulation through growth factors. As a consequence, HSCs proliferate, migrate and secrete enzymes, growth factors and ECM proteins. Several HSC mitogens have been identified. PDGF is a potent mitogen for cultured HSCs and along with its cognate receptor is upregulated during HSC activation [12]. Other identified mitogens include ET-1, IGF, VEGF, FGF, EGF, thrombin, arginine-vasopressin and angiotensin II. One of the most studied growth factors involved in fibrogenesis is TGF-β1, which is an important mediator in the process of fibrogenesis, but with a limited role in HSC activation. At the early phase, TGF-β originates both from platelets and inflammatory cells including Kupffer cells, however, during the perpetuation phase, activated HSCs become its major source. TGF-β1 activates gene transcription and cell release of most ECM components including types I and III collagens, laminin, and fibronectin [13]. HSC activation makes these cells more reactive to TGF-β through the expression or upregulation of the three TGF-β receptors (TGFβR1, TGFβR2, and TGFβR3), specific serine–threonine membrane proteins that activate the Smad signaling pathway. TGF-β can induce apoptosis of epithelial cells including hepatocytes and the consequent impairment of liver regeneration during fibrogenesis [14]. Many other mediators are implicated in liver fibrogenesis. For example, while leptin has a direct stimulatory fibrogenic effect on HSCs, endothelin-1 (ET-1) represents the key contractile stimulus for activated HSCs [15-16]. In fibrotic liver, ET-1 increases and nitric oxide (NO) decreases, shifting the balance towards HSC contraction with consequent modifications of the liver blood flow and portal resistance during fibrosis and cirrhosis [17]. ET-1 is produced in activated HSCs whereas ET-A and ET-B receptors are expressed in quiescent cells [16]. The link between inflammation and fibrosis in liver is bidirectional in a reciprocal crosstalk. HSCs are, for example, directly activated by cytokines, ROS and growth factors and release chemokines or differentiation factors such as monocyte chemotactic protein-1 (MCP-1) and macrophage colony-stimulating factor (M-CSF), thus enhancing the inflammation state. Secretion of cytokines by resident or incoming lymphocytes also contributes to the regulation of fibrogenesis. For example, CD-4 T cells can promote either cell-mediated immunity through secretion of IFN-γ, Il-2 or TNF (Th1 cells) or humoral immunity (Th2 cells) through IL4, IL5, or IL13 secretion. Experimental evidence suggests that different profiles may favor or limit fibrosis. A study has shown that the liver inflammatory background modifies mRNA expression of ADAMTS and TIMP3. In particular, ADAMTS-1 mRNA expression was significantly increased by IL-1β and IL-6 in HepG2 cells. In addition, IL-1β significantly increased ADAMTS-4 mRNA expression in HepG2 cells. However, TIMP3 mRNA expression was downregulated after TNF-α treatment [18]. Inflammatory cells actively take part in proteolysis activation and consequent release of growth factors from ECM, justifying the potential role of the "anti-inflammatory therapy" as a new strategic cancer therapy.

Fibrogenesis Is a Dynamic Process Leading to Fibrosis

Patients with liver chronic disease can be divided into rapid, intermediate, and slow fibrosers according to progression rate. Several host factors contribute to these different phenotypes. In particular, a faster progression rate has been observed in male patients with elevated age at infection time. Other cofactors are alcohol consumption or HIV co-infection. Interestingly, several gene polymorphisms, such as those involving TGF-β and angiotensinogen gene promoters, have been associated with a higher risk of fibrosis development [19]. Dynamism of fibrogenic process should not be seen only in terms of progression. In fact, several studies strongly suggest that regression of fibrosis is possible [20]. In experimental mouse models of fibrosis using chronic carbon tetrachloride (CCl4) intoxication or bile duct ligation, investigators showed that the arrest of fibrogenic stimulus induced spontaneous fibrosis reversion [21]. At cirrhosis stage, regression becomes very difficult but in theory still possible.

MMPs enzymes have a crucial role in ECM remodeling during liver fibrogenesis. Each of these calcium- and zinc-dependent enzymes is specific for an ECM component. While MMP-1 is the key enzyme for fibrillar collagen destruction, MMP-2 and MMP-9 are able to digest basement membrane components. In the early phase of human fibrogenesis, MMP-2 and MMP-9 upregulation and MMP-1 downregulation is observed [22]. Considering that MMP activation is balanced by TIMPs, it is easily deducible that TIMP expression is altered in the fibrogenic process. During progression of liver fibrosis, there is a marked increase in TIMP-1 and TIMP-2 leading to a net decrease in the catalytic activity of MMPs [22-23].

In this dinamic balance between fibrosis progression and regression, HSCs are crucial cellular elements. Activated stellate cells progressively disappear, but whether these cells reverse to a quiescent phenotype or die by apoptosis is still matter of debate. Supporting the hypothesis of apoptosis, there is the evidence that, when activated HSCs transdifferentiate into myofibroblastic phenotype, they express different cell death receptors such as Fas-Fas-ligand and the nerve growth factor receptor. However, an interesting study has recently shown that reversal of activated HSCs towards a more quiescent phenotype contributes to the termination of liver fibrogenesis and fibrosis regression [24]. The inactivated HSCs are similar to quiescent HSCs. Inactivated HSCs express desmin, glial fibrillary acidic protein and synemin, but do not express α-SMA. They also show an increased response to a second fibrogenic stimulus in comparison to quiescent HSCs. In a comparative study between activated and senescent human HSCs, a different expression in cell cycle and proliferation related genes was found [25]. Several factors involved in HSCs senescence have been reported. For example, matricellular protein cysteine-rich protein 61 (CCN1/Cyr61) accumulates in hepatocytes in cirrhosis and, after secretion, induces senescence in activated HSCs and portal fibroblasts [26]. This mechanism, along with the engagement of integrin $\alpha6\beta1$, results in generation of several reactive oxygen species with a consequent antifibrotic gene expression. Immune cells and Natural Killer cells in particular are found in contiguity of the senescent HSCs and thought to clear the senescent HSCs. A very interesting study in this field was that of Klein et al. [27]. In a mouse model of liver fibrosis, these authors demonstrated that atorvastatin, a cholesterol-lowering drug with a recognized effect on liver fibrosis and portal hypertension, induced senescence of activated HSCs. Using senescence marker p21 and beta-galactosidase, HSC marker desmin and myofibroblasts marker α-SMA, these authors observed induction of cell senescence after 5 weeks of bile duct-ligation tretament correlating to the more advanced fibrosis and number of myofibroblasts. This would mean that senescence induction in activated HSCs and myofibroblasts by administration of atorvastatin may lead to promising results during fully established fibrogenesis. Previously, cellular senescence was considered an impediment to carcinogenesis as the direct consequence of stable cell cycle arrest. On the contrary, a recent surprising discovery has unvailed that senescent cells can produce a large variety of pro-inflammatory signaling proteins and cytokines with promoting effects on tumor growth, the so-called senescence-associated secretory phenotype. Yoshimoto et al. induced HCC in p21-p-luciferase (p21Waf1/Cip1) bearing neonatal mice after administration of a chemical carcinogen and a high-fat diet. The importance of senescent cells was demonstrated considering that HCC developed without liver fibrosis and so the origin of senescent HSCs was not caused by liver fibrosis [28]. On one hand, senescence of HSCs contains progression of fibrosis. On the other hand, it may induce proliferation and neoplastic transformation of hepatocytes in chronic liver disease, so that senescent HSCs may represent an interesting target for developing new therapeutic strategies. In this field, other studies will be necessary to better understand the role of inactivated HSCs in the tumor-stroma crosstalk and during cancer progression.

From Fibrosis to Cancer

Many evidences indicate that HCC risk correlate with degree of fibrosis. In a Japanese cohort of HCV patients, the risk of cirrhotic patients (F4) was 5.8% per patient per year, which was much higher than those patients who had less fibrosis (F1-F3, 0.5-2.6%) [29]. The mechanisms linking the fibrotic process to the development of HCC remain largely unknown. The risk for HCC could be reduced through the abrogation of the initial inflammatory insult. However, persistent inflammation and fibrosis eventually represent a real carcinogenic risk. Potential mechanisms of fibrosis-dependent carcinogenesis include: i) increased integrin signaling by ECM proteins; ii) paracrine signaling between hepatic stromal cells and hepatocytes; iii) increased stromal stiffness; iv) growth factor sequestration by ECM; v) reduced tumor surveillance by immune cells such as NK and NKT [30]. In liver fibrosis, the enhanced deposition of fibronectin and fibrillar collagen types I and III causes cellular responses through engagement of integrins. Integrins are transmembrane receptors that promote cell growth and survival by activating the PI3K and MAPK signaling cascades [31]. Another proposed mechanism for integrin-mediated carcinogenesis includes increased migration and anti-apoptotic signaling. As mentioned above, activated HSCs produce factors that stimulate tumor cell proliferation and angiogenesis such as growth factors and cytokines. Tumors may in turn signal to recruit stromal cells. For example, tumor secretion of PDGF and TGF-β stimulates myofibroblast activation and recruitment. The hedgehog pathway is another example of mediators of tumor-stroma interactions in the liver. Elevated hedgehog signaling that are associated with liver injury promotes liver regeneration and tumor formation. The tumorigenic effect of hedgehog is supposed to be mediated by an increase in myofibroblasts activity and fibrosis [32]. Elevated stiffness of the liver evaluated by transient elastography is correlated with a higher risk of HCC [33] and stromal stiffness could have an early influence in HCC development. It has been demonstrated that a stiff collagen gel inhibits differentiation and promotes proliferation of primary hepatocyte [34]. In agreement with these observations, it has been proposed that an increase in ECM stiffness in fibrotic liver promotes HSCs activation and a positive feedback loop that continues to enhance fibrosis.

Growth factors such as FGF and TGF-β are embedded in the ECM. In the ECM, TGF-β is bound to the latent TGF-β binding proteins (LTBPs), and in this form TGF-β is unable to signal. This suggests that ECM accumulation of this factor may lead to increased proliferation and decreased apoptosis, since the TGF-β signaling axis is a suppressor of cell proliferation. However, in the setting of inflammation, elevated MMP activity can release matrix-embedded TGF-β. The fibrotic ECM contains elevated concentrations of embedded TGF-β and releases greater amounts of the cytokine that exerts the overall effect of inhibiting proliferation and promoting apoptosis. NK cells induce apoptosis in cells with downregulated expression of class I major histocompatability complex or with up-regulated stress-induced ligands. In addition to being involved in tumor cells killing, NK cells down-regulate the fibrogenic process through induction of apoptosis of activated HSCs. It is not a coincidence that in chronic liver disease NK cells have reduced activity. In fact, fibrosis, that represents a mechanical barrier, may impede the contact of NK cells with their cell targets and therefore their proper function [35]. It would be interesting to understand whether the composition of ECM differs depending on the etiology and if the overall changes in ECM composition are necessary to stimulate HCC formation and progression or it is sufficient the change of a single ECM component at a specific cut-off level. Several immunohistochemical studies indicated that the distribution of ECM components such as fibronectin, laminin and collagen IV in HCC reflects the differentiation of the tumor. Differentiated tumors show a relatively intact basement membrane whereas poorly differentiated tumors are marked with a more defective basement membrane composition. Comparing small *versus* large liver cell dysplasia similar differences can be noticed, considering that liver cell dysplasia is characterized by an abnormal tenascin and type IV collagen expression. Fang et al. showed that type IV collagen degradation and ECM remodelling is a continuous process necessary for cancer cells invasion [36]. Another recent study by Lai et al., using two different mouse models, has characterized proteomic changes occurring in liver fibrosis, steatosis and HCC. In particular, these authors identified twenty-six collagen-encoding genes expressing 16 collagens and described important alterations at the post-transcriptional protein level for six collagens and lysine hydroxylation changes for 14 collagens. The result was the identification of new ECM and integrin components, new crosstalks between ECM and cancer, relevant for HCC classification, diagnosis, prevention or therapy [37]. From all these studies, it is becoming clear that there is a continuous matrix remodelling and dynamic change in ECM and these findings could have a clinical impact. For example, fibril-forming type I and type III collagens are predominant in HCC, so they could be potentially used as serum markers for liver fibrosis assessment (i.e. the Enhanced Liver Fibrosis – ELF score) [38].

Vascularization

Changes in the perisinusoidal space or space of Disse is a common early complication observed during liver fibrosis that implyies the accumulation of collagen types I and III and the formation of a framework of fibrillar collagens which replace the basement membrane material. These matrix changes are associated with modifications of sinusoidal cells including the loss of pores of endothelial cells, a process known as "sinusoid capillarization."

Approximately 95% of the liver's oxygenated blood comes from the portal vein. In contrast, about 80% of oxygenated blood for HCCs comes from hepatic arterial branches. This HCC hypervascular pattern so different from the normal liver vascularization represents the rational for using enhanced imaging techniques to diagnose HCC and for using of therapeutic approaches such as transarterial chemoembolization (TACE) and antiangiogenetic agents.

Angiogenesis

Rarely an avascular tumor grows more than 2–3 mm, but after becoming vascularized, the progression is rapid. It is now widely accepted that the switch to the angiogenic phenotype involves both the upregulation of angiogenic stimulators and the downregulation of inhibitors. Various signals such as metabolic and mechanical stress, inflammation, and genetic alteration trigger this switch. Vascular endothelial growth factor (VEGF) and angiopoietins are the most studied among the different angiogenic factors and shown to work sinergically. Increased VEGF expression has been shown in HCC and high VEGF expression is associated with high proliferative index, poor encapsulation, portal vein thrombosis, microscopic venous invasion and poor prognosis after resection [39-40]. Peritumoral liver tissue is usually inflamed and angiogenic. Cirrhotic liver show a higher VEGF expression compared with normal liver. Several factors are involved in VEGF expression. In hypoxic tissues, the transcription complex HIF-1A plays a major role in inducing the transcription of VEGF. Other factors involved in VEGF upregulation are exposure to growth factors such as EGF, TGF and IL-1, suppression of the p53 or von Hippel-Lindau tumor-suppressor genes and mutations or amplification of the RAS oncogene. Recently, angiopoietins (Ang) have been identified as a group of ligands of the tyrosine kinase Tie-2 receptor, localized to the vascular endothelial cells. The Tie-2 signal pathway is defined through the quantitative balance of activities between Ang-1, the agonist, and Ang-2, the antagonist. Unlike VEGFs, angiopoietins do not induce proliferation, migration, or tubule formation, but they are involved in the sprouting of vascular endothelial cells. Various studies have revealed that angiopoietin-1 promotes the stabilization and tightening of developing vessels by mediating the interaction between endothelial cells and smooth muscle cells/pericytes. Instead, angiopoietin-2 induces vascular destabilization by blocking angiopoietin-1 signaling. Accordingly, in the hypervascular type of HCC, angiopoietin-2 is upregulated and promotes a vigorous angiogenic response in the presence of VEGF or vessel regression in the absence of VEGF [41]. In contrast, angiopoietin-2 is not expressed in normal hepatocytes, which express angiopoietin-1. Considering that both cirrhotic livers and well-differentiated HCCs show high VEGF levels, authors have proposed the reversal expression of angiopoietin-1 and -2 as the key signal to the angiogenic switch in HCC [42].

Other angiogenic factors described include basic fibroblast growth factor, transforming growth factor-β, insulin growth factor-2R, platelet-derived endothelial cell growth factor, tissue factor and cyclooxygenase- 2.

References

[1] Goldenberg D, Ayesh S, Schneider T, Pappo O, Jurim O, Eid A, Fellig Y, Dadon T, Ariel I, de Groot N, Hochberg A, Galun E. 2002. "Analysis of differentially expressed genes in hepatocellular carcinoma using cDNA arrays." *Mol Carcinog* 33:113-24.

[2] Coulouarn C, Corlu A, Glaise D, Guénon I, Thorgeirsson SS, and Clément B. 2012. "Hepatocyte-stellate cell cross-talk in the liver engenders a permissive inflammatory microenvironment that drives progression in hepatocellular carcinoma." *Cancer Res* 72:2533-42. Accessed March 14, 2012. doi: 10.1158/0008-5472.

[3] Amann T, Bataille F, Spruss T, Mühlbauer M, Gäbele E, Schölmerich J, Kiefer P, Bosserhoff AK, and Hellerbrand C. 2009. "Activated hepatic stellate cells promote tumorigenicity of hepatocellular carcinoma." *Cancer Sci* 100:646-53. Accessed January 21, 2009. doi: 10.1111/ j.1349-7006.2009.01087.

[4] Mazzocca A, Dituri F, Lupo L, Quaranta M, Antonaci S, and Giannelli G. 2011. "Tumor-secreted lysophostatidic acid accelerates hepatocellular carcinoma progression by promoting differentiation of peritumoral fibroblasts in myofibroblasts." *Hepatology* 54:920-30. Accessed August 8, 2011. doi: 10.1002 /hep.24485.

[5] D.S.R. Lockwood, D.C. Gotley. 2005. "Interaction of tumor with host stroma in hepatocellular carcinoma." In *Integration/ Interaction of Oncologic Growth,* edited by Gary G. Meadows, 165-176. Springer Netherlands.

[6] Ng IO, Lai EC, Ng MM, Fan ST. 1992. "Tumor encapsulation in hepatocellular carcinoma. A pathologic study of 189 cases." *Cancer* 70:45-9.

[7] Mazzocca A, Fransvea E, Dituri F, Lupo L, Antonaci S, Giannelli G. 2010. "Down-regulation of connective tissue growth factor by inhibition of transforming growth factor beta blocks the tumor-stroma cross-talk and tumor progression in hepatocellular carcinoma." *Hepatology* 51:523-34.

[8] Yu Q, Stamenkovic I. 2000. "Cell surface-localized matrix metalloproteinase-9 proteolytically activates TGF-beta and promotes tumor invasion and angiogenesis." *Genes Dev* 14:163-76.

[9] Svegliati Baroni G, D'Ambrosio L, Ferretti G, Casini A, Di Sario A, Salzano R, Ridolfi F, Saccomanno S, Jezequel AM, Benedetti A. 1998. "Fibrogenic effect of oxidative stress on rat hepatic stellate cells." *Hepatology* 27:720-6.

[10] Paradis V, Mathurin P, Kollinger M, Imbert-Bismut F, Charlotte F, Piton A, Opolon P, Holstege A, Poynard T, Bedossa P. 1997. "In situ detection of lipid peroxidation in chronic hepatitis C: correlation with pathological features." *J Clin Pathol* 50:401-6.

[11] Jarnagin WR, Rockey DC, Koteliansky VE, Wang SS, Bissell DM. 1994. "Expression of variant fibronectins in wound healing: cellular source and biological activity of the EIIIA segment in rat hepatic fibrogenesis." *J Cell Biol* 127:2037-48.

[12] Pinzani M, Gesualdo L, Sabbah GM, Abboud HE. 1989. "Effects of platelet-derived growth factor and other polypeptide mitogens on DNA synthesis and growth of cultured rat liver fat-storing cells." *J Clin Invest* 84:1786-93.

[13] Casini A, Pinzani M, Milani S, Grappone C, Galli G, Jezequel AM, Schuppan D, Rotella CM, Surrenti C. 1993. "Regulation of extracellular matrix synthesis by transforming growth factor β-1 in human fat storing cells." *Gastroenterology* 105:245-53.

[14] Kim BC, Mamura M, Choi KS, Calabretta B, Kim SJ. 2002. "Transforming growth factor beta 1 induces apoptosis through cleavage of BAD in a Smad3-dependent mechanism in FaO hepatoma cells." *Mol Cell Biol* 22:1369-78.

[15] Ikejima K, Takei Y, Honda H, Hirose M, Yoshikawa M, Zhang YJ, Lang T, Fukuda T, Yamashina S, Kitamura T, Sato N. 2002. "Leptin receptor-mediated signaling regulates hepatic fibrogenesis and remodeling of extracellular matrix in the rat." *Gastroenterology* 122: 1399-410.

[16] Housset C, Rockey DC, Bissell DM. 1993. "Endothelin receptors in rat liver: lipocytes as a contractile target for endothelin 1." *Proc Natl Acad Sci U S A* 90: 9266-70.

[17] Kawada N, Tran-Thi TA, Klein H, Decker K. 1993. "The contraction of hepatic stellate (Ito) cells stimulated with vasoactive substances. Possible involvement ofendothelin 1 and nitric oxide in the regulation of the sinusoidal tonus." *Eur J Biochem* 213:815-23.

[18] Turner SL, Mangnall D, Bird NC, Bunning RA, Blair-Zajdel ME. 2012. "Expression of ADAMTS-1, ADAMTS-4, ADAMTS-5 and TIMP3 by hepatocellular carcinoma cell lines." *Int J Oncol* 41:1043-9.

[19] Powell EE, Edwards-Smith CJ, Hay JL, Clouston AD, Crawford DH, Shorthouse C, Purdie DM, Jonsson JR. 2000. "Host genetic factors influence disease progression in chronic hepatitis C." *Hepatology* 31:828-33.

[20] Wanless IR, Nakashima E, Sherman M. 2000. "Regression of human cirrhosis. Morphologic features and the genesis of incomplete septal cirrhosis." *Arch Pathol Lab Med* 124:1599-607.

[21] Iredale JP, Benyon RC, Pickering J, McCullen M, Northrop M, Pawley S, Hovell C, Arthur MJ. 1998. "Mechanisms of spontaneous resolution of rat liver fibrosis. Hepatic stellate cell apoptosis and reduced hepatic expression of metalloproteinase inhibitors." *J Clin Invest* 102:538-49.

[22] Iredale JP, Benyon RC, Arthur MJ, Ferris WF, Alcolado R, Winwood PJ, Clark N, Murphy G. 1996. "Tissue inhibitor of metalloproteinase-1 messenger RNA expression is enhanced relative to interstitial collagenase messenger RNA in experimental liver injury and fibrosis." *Hepatology* 24:176-84.

[23] Benyon RC, Iredale JP, Goddard S, Winwood PJ, Arthur MJ. 1996. "Expression of tissue inhibitor of metalloproteinases 1 and 2 is increased in fibrotic human liver." *Gastroenterology* 110:821-31.

[24] Krizhanovsky V, Yon M, Dickins RA, Hearn S, Simon J, Miething C, Yee H, Zender L, Lowe SW. 2008. "Senescence of activated stellate cells limits liver fibrosis." *Cell* 134:657-67.

[25] Schnabl B, Purbeck CA, Choi YH, Hagedorn CH, Brenner D. 2003. "Replicative senescence of activated human hepatic stellate cells is accompanied by a pronounced inflammatory but less fibrogenic phenotype." *Hepatology* 37: 653-64.

[26] Kim KH, Chen CC, Monzon RI, Lau LF. 2013. "Matricellular protein CCN1 promotes regression of liver fibrosis through induction of cellular senescence in hepatic myofibroblasts." *Mol Cell Biol* 33:2078-90.

[27] Klein S, Klösel J, Schierwagen R, Körner C, Granzow M, Huss S, Mazar IG, Weber S, van den Ven PF, Pieper-Fürst U, Fürst DO, Nattermann J, Lammert F,Sauerbruch T, Trebicka J. 2012. "Atorvastatin inhibits proliferation and apoptosis, but induces senescence in hepatic myofibroblasts and thereby attenuates hepatic fibrosis in rats." *Lab Invest* 92:1440-50.

[28] Yoshimoto S, Loo TM, Atarashi K, Kanda H, Sato S, Oyadomari S, Iwakura Y, Oshima K, Morita H, Hattori M, Honda K, Ishikawa Y, Hara E, and Ohtani N. 2013. "Obesity-induced gut microbial metabolite promotes liver cancer through senescence secretome." *Nature* 499:97-101. Accessed June 26, 2013. doi: 10.1038/nature12347.

[29] Kiyosawa K. 2002. "Trend of liver cirrhosis as precancerous lesions." In *Hepatol Res,* edited by Kiyosawa K, 24:S40-45. Elsevier Science.

[30] Zhang DY, Friedman SL. 2012. "Fibrosis-Dependent Mechanisms of Hepatocarcinogenesis." *Hepatology* 56:769-75.

[31] Cox D, Brennan M, Moran N. 2010. "Integrins as therapeutic targets: lessons and opportunities." *Nat Rev Drug Discov* 9:804-20.

[32] Ochoa B, Syn WK, Delgado I, Karaca GF, Jung Y, Wang J, Zubiaga AM, Fresnedo O, Omenetti A, Zdanowicz M, Choi SS, Diehl AM. 2010. "Hedgehog signaling is critical for normal liver regeneration after partial hepatectomy in mice." *Hepatology* 51:1712-23.

[33] Masuzaki R, Tateishi R, Yoshida H, Yoshida H, Sato S, Kato N, Kanai F, Sugioka Y, Ikeda H, Shiina S, Kawabe T, Omata M. 2008. "Risk assessment of hepatocellular carcinoma in chronic hepatitis C patients by transient elastography." *J Clin Gastroenterol* 42:839-43.

[34] Hansen LK, Wilhelm J, Fassett JT. 2006. "Regulation of hepatocyte cell cycle progression and differentiation by type I collagen structure." *Curr Top Dev Biol* 72: 205-36.

[35] Kawarabayashi N, Seki S, Hatsuse K, Ohkawa T, Koike Y, Aihara T, Habu Y, Nakagawa R, Ami K, Hiraide H, Mochizuki H. 2000. "Decrease of CD56þT cells and natural killer cells in cirrhotic livers with hepatitis C may be involved in their susceptibility to hepatocellular carcinoma." *Hepatology* 32:962-9.

[36] Fang M, Yuan JP, Peng CW, Pang DW, and Li Y. 2013. "Quantum dots-based in situ molecular imaging of dynamic changes of collagen IV during cancer invasion." *Biomaterials* 34:8708-17. Accessed August 9, 2013. doi: 10.1016/j. biomaterials.2013.07.069.

[37] Lai KK, Shang S, Lohia N, Booth GC, Masse DJ, Fausto N, Campbell JS, and Beretta L. 2011. "Extracellular matrix dynamics in hepatocarcinogenesis: a comparative proteomics study of PDGFC transgenic and Pten null mouse models." *PLoS Genet* 7:e1002147. Accessed June 23, 2011. doi: 10.1371/ journal.pgen.1002147.

[38] Rosenberg WM, Voelker M, Thiel R, Becka M, Burt A, Schuppan D, Hubscher S, Roskams T, Pinzani M, Arthur MJ. 2004. "European Liver

Fibrosis Group. Serum markers detect the presence of liver fibrosis: a cohort study." *Gastroenterology* 127:1704-13.
[39] Chow NH, Hsu PI, Lin XZ, Yang HB, Chan SH, Cheng KS, Huang SM, Su IJ. 1997. "Expression of vascular endothelial growth factor in normal liver and hepatocellular carcinoma: an immunohistochemical study." *Hum Pathol* 28:698-703.
[40] Poon RT, Ng IO, Lau C, Zhu LX, Yu WC, Lo CM, Fan ST, Wong J. 2001. "Serum vascular endothelial growth factor predicts venous invasion in hepatocellular carcinoma: a prospective study." *Ann Surg* 233:227-35.
[41] Holash J, Maisonpierre PC, Compton D, Boland P, Alexander CR, Zagzag D, Yancopoulos GD, Wiegand SJ. 1999. "Vessel cooption, regression, and growth in tumors mediated by angiopoietins and VEGF." *Science* 284:1994-8.
[42] Sugimachi K, Tanaka S, Terashi T, Taguchi K, Rikimaru T, Sugimachi K. 2002. "The mechanisms of angiogenesis in hepatocellular carcinoma: angiogenic switch during tumor progression." *Surgery* 131:S135-41.

Chapter 5

HCC Heterogeneity

HCC is characterized by a great heterogeneity in terms of cancer behavior, progression and response to therapy, so it could be considered not a single entity rather a variety of different cancers. This high level of heterogeneity could be explained considering the number of genetic, epigenetic and environmental factors and several cellular and molecular pathways involved. It has been proposed that the most frequent gene aberrations observed in HCCs may arise from the selection of alleles from a randomly mixture of altered genes supporting survival and growth advantages. This has been reported by a recent study describing the presence of distinct diagnostic signatures derived from different biopsies of the same tumor [1]. However, HCC heterogeneity is not only the manifestation of the genetic or epigenetic heterogeneity. As the natural history of disease indicates, the cellular-type involved has also a relevant clinical impact. Different cancer cell types could be the initial transformed cells and a different prevalence of cancer-like stem cells has been described in HCC. Another factor to consider is the hepatic microenvironment. According to the different etiologies of cirrhosis and the several host factors involved, liver cancer behavior and progression largely vary from cancer to cancer in patients. As explained above, there is a continuous crosstalk between cancer cells and microenvironment with reciprocal influence. On one hand, it is possible to study the effect of the stromal components on the cancer cell signaling pathways. One method is to stimulate cancer cells with stromal cell-secreted cytokines, growth factors, or soluble ECM. On the other hand, it is possible to analyze the profiles of secreted cytokines in cancer cells, which seems to be quite specific. For example, the screening of secretome in HCC cell lines has revealed that each cell line has specific clusters of secreted proteins involved in several activities such as metabolism, cytoskeleton/mobility, protein synthesis and degradation, transport, DNA replication, gene regulation, cell cycle and transduction pathways [2]. Therefore, this could significantly contribute to the HCC heterogeneity.

However, limitations or major obstacles in these studies are represented by the usage of cell lines *versus* primary isolated stromal cells and the usage of nude mouse models, which partly reflect the immunological pattern and the microenvironment present in human HCC. Important improvements in screening, subtyping and categorizing HCC have been obtained by using the so called "omics signatures." The identification of specific genomic signatures would have important clinical impact in terms on prediction, phenotyping and targeted terapies. For example, in a study by Boyault and collaborators, the HCCs were classified into six subgroups according to their clinical and genetic characteristics. These authors demonstrated that half of tumors were characterized by active WNT or AKT signaling pathways that could be potential therapeutic targets [3]. Wurmbach et al., analyzing the multistep-carcinogenesis in HCV patients, identified gene signatures specific for each stage of progress [4]. The relevance of this study was the identification of a 186-gene expression signature specific for the overall death in HCV patients who underwent surgery treatment for HCC. This signature is also a sensitive predictor of poor outcome in patients with newly diagnosed HCV-related early-stage cirrhosis, identifying those patients at risk of HCC development [5]. Moreover, Divella et al. demonstrated that tumor heterogeneity is closely linked with inflammation, suggesting the presence of two distinct pathogenic mechanisms in HCC development depending on whether the etiology is viral or nonviral [6]. These authors observed that the frequency of the 4G/4G genotype was significantly higher in HCC patients co-infected with HBV and HCV than in those without viral infection and this genotype was also related with elevated plasma levels of SERPINE1.

References

[1] Gerlinger M, Rowan AJ, Horswell S, Larkin J, Endesfelder D, Gronroos E, Martinez P, Matthews N, Stewart A, Tarpey P, Varela I, Phillimore B, Begum S,McDonald NQ, Butler A, Jones D, Raine K, Latimer C, Santos CR, Nohadani M, Eklund AC, Spencer-Dene B, Clark G, Pickering L,

Stamp G, Gore M, Szallasi Z,Downward J, Futreal PA, Swanton C. 2012. "Intratumor heterogeneity and branched evolution revealed by multiregion sequencing." *N Engl J Med* 366: 883-92.

[2] Srisomsap C, Sawangareetrakul P, Subhasitanont P, Chokchaichamnankit D, Chiablaem K, Bhudhisawasdi V, Wongkham S, and Svasti J. 2010. "Proteomic studies of cholangiocarcinoma and hepatocellular carcinoma cell secretomes." *J Biomed Biotechnol* 2010:437143. Accessed December 27, 2009.doi: 10.1155/ 2010/437143.

[3] Boyault S, Rickman DS, de Reyniès A, Balabaud C, Rebouissou S, Jeannot E, Hérault A, Saric J, Belghiti J, Franco D, Bioulac-Sage P, Laurent-Puig P,Zucman-Rossi J. 2007. "Transcriptome classification of HCC is related to gene alterations and to new therapeutic targets." *Hepatology* 45:42-52.

[4] Wurmbach E, Chen YB, Khitrov G, Zhang W, Roayaie S, Schwartz M, Fiel I, Thung S, Mazzaferro V, Bruix J, Bottinger E, Friedman S, Waxman S, Llovet JM. 2007. "Genome-wide molecular profiles of HCV-induced dysplasia and hepatocellular carcinoma." *Hepatology* 45:938-47.

[5] Hoshida Y, Villanueva A, Sangiovanni A, Sole M, Hur C, Andersson KL, Chung RT, Gould J, Kojima K, Gupta S, Taylor B, Crenshaw A, Gabriel S, Minguez B,Iavarone M, Friedman SL, Colombo M, Llovet JM, and Golub TR. 2013. "Prognostic gene expression signature for patients with hepatitis C-related early-stage cirrhosis." *Gastroenterology* 144:1024-30. Accessed January 17, 2013. doi: 10.1053/j.gastro.2013.01. 021.

[6] Divella R, Mazzocca A, Gadaleta C, Simone G, Paradiso A, Quaranta M, Daniele A. 2012. "Influence of plasminogen activator inhibitor-1 (SERPINE1) 4G/5G polymorphism on circulating SERPINE-1 antigen expression in HCC associated with viral infection." *Cancer Genomics Proteomics* 9:193-8.

Chapter 6

Clinical Aspects of HCC: The Screening

A better understanding of the natural history and the pathobiology of HCC in the last two decades, has promoted implementation of surveillance programs of risk patients to diagnose HCC at an early stage and improved prognosis and therapeutic approaches to these patients.

Liver Fibrosis Screening

Liver biopsy is considered the gold standard for fibrosis assessment but it has several limitations including significant morbidity, observer variation dependent on the pathologist experience, the scoring system used and the heterogeneous distribution of fibrosis in the liver tissue. Image analysis is sensitive, however, it is able to estimate only the amount of ECM deposited. For this reason, scoring systems are useful to take into account features like architectural distortion and topographical distribution. Well-defined semiquantitative scores are the Metavir score or the Knodell index. Recently, the use of several biomarkers derived from ECM molecules (hyaluronan, P-III-P, MMPs, TIMP) or a composite index made by association of several markers of liver function has been proposed for fibrosis staging [1-2]. Proteomic analysis and powerful imaging techniques should lead to further progress.

HCC Clinical Presentation

The clinical presentation of HCC is mainly determined by the degree of liver dysfunction and the tumor burden, which depends on the "timing" of diagnosis. In Western countries and Japan, thanks to the implementation of surveillance programs for patients with high risk, HCC is frequently diagnosed at an early asymptomatic stage. On the contrary, HCCs arising in a non-cirrhotic liver usually are detected outside surveillance programs and exhibit a rapid and infiltrative growth with frequent vascular invasion and metastases, likely due to delayed diagnosis. In Italy, 45% of HCCs developing in chronic liver diseases are diagnosed under surveillance in preclinical phase and over 55% of HCCs detected under surveillance are cancers in non-advanced stages, however, this percentage becomes one third for the HCCs diagnosed outside surveillance [3]. Symptoms and signs commonly present are abdominal pain/discomfort, hepatomegaly, jaundice, ascites and constitutional syndrome (fatigue, malaise, fever and weight loss). Less common are digestive or peritoneal bleeding and hepatic encephalopathy. For a complete clinical evaluation of a patient with HCC, the history is very important to evaluate any predisposing conditions such as hepatitis, metabolic syndrome, blood transfusion, intravenous drugs or alchool abuse. A family history of HCC or hepatitis should be investigated as well as the social history including job descriptions for industrial exposure to possible carcinogens. Physical examination should include assessing clinical signs of underlying liver disease such as jaundice, ascites, peripheral edema, spider nevi, palmar erythema, weight loss and splenomegaly. Laboratory tests should include blood count, liver function tests (i.e. bilirubin, albumin, gamma-glutamyl transpeptidase, alkaline phosphatase, transaminases, prothrombin time, ammoniemia), serum protein electrophoresis, cholinesterase and cholesterol, renal function tests (i.e. urea, creatinine and electrolytes), serum and tissue iron levels, tumor markers, and HBV and HCV serology.

HCC Imaging

As mentioned above, screening in HCC patients is important to diagnose HCC at early stages, when more effective therapies are possible, considering that almost 50% of HCCs detected under surveillance are susceptible to effective therapy [4]. Consensus screening recommendations advise that abdominal ultrasound should be performed every 6–12 months for patients with diseases at risk for HCC.

Zhang and coworkers evaluated the efficacy of surveillance strategies of AFP plus ultrasonography every 6 months in patients with hepatitis B (HBV) and compared to a cohort of patients who did not receive any surveillance. These authors demonstrated that the screening program reduces overall mortality and allows diagnosis at earlier stages when more therapy choises are possible [5]. In addition, a meta-analysis by Singal and collaborators showed that ultrasonography was a surveillance strategy with a sensitivity of 63% to diagnose early stage HCC in cirrhotic patients, and ultrasonography every 6 months showed a higher sensitivity for early HCC than ultrasonography every 12 months [6].

Frequently, HCC diagnosis is solely established by imaging criteria. These criteria are based on the CT or MRI contrast enhancement pattern with an intense contrast uptake by tumor mass in the arterial phase followed by contrast washout in the venous delayed phase. This typical vascular pattern is known as "the HCC radiological hallmark." If HCC displays characteristic appearance, biopsy is not necessary. However, atypical vascular lesions always require biopsy. Liver biopsy has the benefits of certain diagnosis, but it has several risks such as bleeding and the hazard of tumor "seeding" into the biopsy needle track. MRI differentiates regenerative nodules in cirrhotic livers more accurately than CT. The recent introduction of new MRI imaging agents has proved very useful for detection of small lesions. It has been reported that gadoxetic acid-enhanced MRI and DWI have a high sensitivity for HCC less than 2 cm in size (91–93%) [7]. An interesting study evaluating patients with cirrhosis and liver nodules with hepatobiliary-specific MRI contrast, multidetector CT, and nodules biopsy showed that MRI was more sensitive and specific for small HCC (<2 cm) than MDCT [8]. According to the recall policy proposed by EASL [9], tumor size is a parameter for screening approach. For nodules ≤1 cm, if stable, a repeated ultrasound is recommended every 4 months for the first year and afterwards every 6 months. In case of growing nodule, it is recomended to evaluate according to its size. For indeterminate 1-2 cm nodules, a 4-phase CT and a dynamic contrast enhanced MRI are recommended in order to point out the radiological hallmark. Diagnosis for these nodules requires two imaging tecniques positive for the presence of the HCC radiological hallmark or only one positive imaging in centers of excellence in the radiology field. Nevertheless, histology is necessary in most of cases, in consideration that the typical vascular pattern occurs in a small proportion of these patients. In tumors greater than 2 cm in diameter, HCC diagnosis can be validated by a single imaging technique (4-phase CT or dynamic contrast enhanced MRI) positive for the HCC radiological hallmark. In case of atypical vascular pattern, liver biopsy is necessary. Biopsy sensitivity is 70-90% depending on tumor size, location, and local experience [10]. Therefore, it is strongly recommended that biopses of small lesions should be evaluated by expert pathologists, and in case of inconclusive biopsies, close follow-up with US every 4 months is highly recommended.

CT or MRI scan should be performed to obtain pre-therapy assessment of the tumor, dimension and number evaluation, location within the liver, proximity to main vessels, identification of portal vein invasion or thrombosis, presence of cirrhosis and ascites (Figure 7-9). Adequate staging of HCC patients should also include a chest CT scan, a brain CT, if neurologic symptoms are present and routine serologic tests. Angiography has almost disappeared from the clinical practice.

Table 2. Recommendations for screening and diagnosis of HCC. Screening is recommended for patients with a liver disease at risk of HCC. For nodules < 1 cm it is recommended to repeat ultrasonography every 4 months the first year and after every 6 months. For nodules > 2 cm 1 positive imaging tecnique is necessary for diagnosis. Diagnosis for nodules 1-2 cm requires 2 positive imaging. It could be sufficient one positive imaging tecnique only in centers of excellence.* In case of nodules with atypical vascular pattern biopsy is necessary

Liver disease at risk of HCC	Abdominal ultrasound+AFP	Every 6-12 months
Nodule <1cm	Repeat US	Every 4-6 months
1 cm<Nodule<2 cm	1* or 2 imaging (CT/MRI) positive for the HCC radiological hallmark If negative biopsy	
Nodule >2 cm	1 imaging (CT or MRI) positive for the HCC radiological hallmark If negative biopsy	

Figure 7. (Continued)

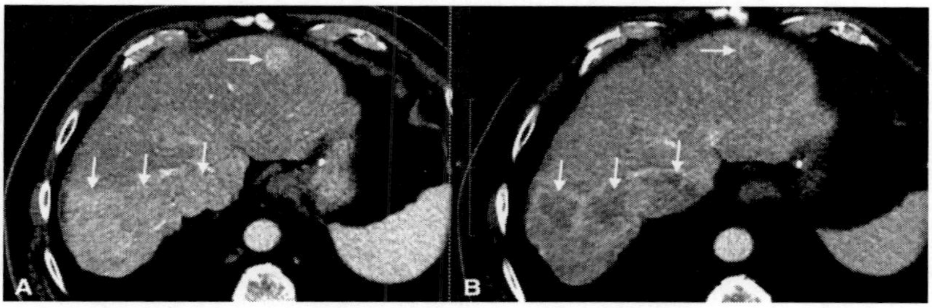

Figure 7. Patient with multifocal infiltrative HCC. Contrast CT in arterial phase (A) and in venous phase (B). The CT highlights a diffuse neoplastic inflitration of the right lobe and in a small nodule of the left lobe (arrows). The nodules are hypervascularised in the arterial phase and hypodense in the venous phase. Image courtesy of Dr. Arnaldo Scardapane, University of Bari.

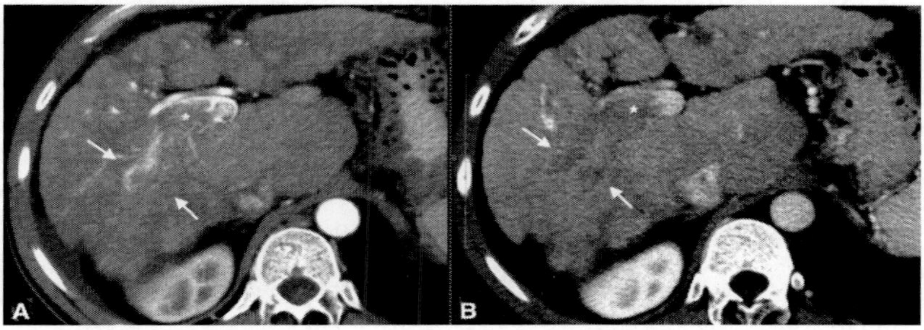

Figure 8. Patient with HCC of the right lobe and neoplastic thrombosis of the portal vein. Contrast CT in arterial phase (A) and in venous phase (B). The CT highlights a diffuse neoplastic infiltration of the right lobe (arrows) with a bulky neoplastic thrombus vegetating in the portal vein (*). Image courtesy of Dr. Arnaldo Scardapane, University of Bari.

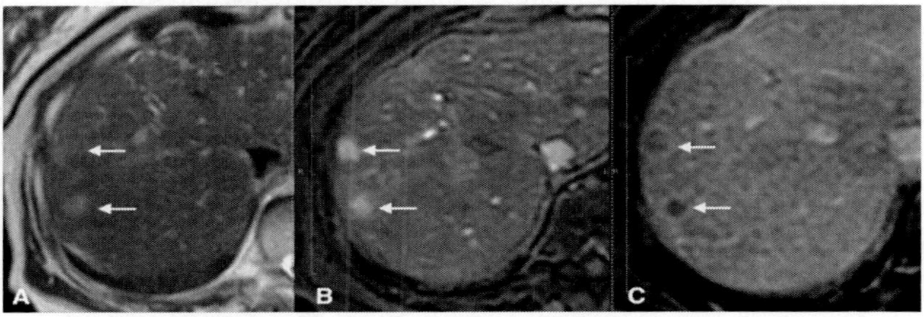

Figure 9. Patient with two nodules of HCC in the VII segment. MR T2 weighted image A), Contrast MR T1 image in arterial phase B) and venous phase C). The MR highlights in the VII segment of the liver two nodules hyperintense in the T2 weighted sequences, that, after contrast enhancement, are shown hypervascularized in the arterial phase and hypointense in the venous phase (arrows). Image courtesy of Dr. Arnaldo Scardapane, University of Bari.

HCC Biomarkers

Serum alpha-fetoprotein (AFP) is a commonly used screening biomarker in patients at risk for HCC, but it has important limits in terms of sensitivity and specificity. In fact, elevated AFP levels can also occur in association with hepatitis without HCC, but levels > 400 ng/ml may indicate the presence of HCC. About 50% of patients with HCC do not have elevations of AFP levels, therefore normal values do not exclude HCC.

Lens culinaris agglutinin (LCA)-reactive AFP (AFP-L3) is an isoform of AFP that has been shown to be highly specific for HCC and may improve the detection of small HCCs [11]. Furthermore, AFP-L3, compared to the total AFP, is superior in HCC diagnosis and prognosis prediction.

Another proposed HCC marker is Descarboxyprothrombin (DCP) also known as protein induced by vitamin K absence or antagonist-II (PIVKA-II). DCP production in HCC cells derives from a post-translational carboxylation defect of the prothrombin precursor. PIVKA-II has a higher specificity for HCC than AFP but is less sensitive. Serum PIVKA-II levels are elevated in about 50–60% of HCC patients but elevated levels of this marker are found only in 15–30% of patients with HCC < 3 cm [12]. Combined use of AFP and PIVKA-II has been proposed to increase the sensitivity and specificity for HCC diagnosis [13].

Glypican-3 (GPC3) is considered a novel tumor marker of HCC that has been widely studied. GPC3 is a heparan sulfate proteoglycan anchored to the plasma membrane which functions as modulator of several growth factors activities. GPC3 is detectable in serum in 40–53% of HCC patients, whereas it is not present in the serum of healthy subjects. Combination of GPC3 and AFP increases the sensitivity in diagnosis without reducing the specificity. Moreover, soluble GPC3 (sGPC3) that is the NH2-terminal portion of GPC3 seems to be more predictive compared to AFP in detection of well or moderately differentiated HCCs.

A check-up of three tumor markers every 6 months has been proposed for HCC screening in Japan, including alpha-fetoprotein, AFP-L3, (measured when AFP is above 20 ng/ml or in the presence of liver mass) and DCP. In combination with these markers, abdominal ultrasonography is done about every 3 months for cirrhotic patients and about every 6 months for patients with chronic hepatitis. If HCC is suspected, a dynamic computed tomography is performed.

An autoantibody signature or humoral response against oncoproteins has been described in HCC patients and might be used as an accurate screening test. Also, the recent identification of HCC progenitor cells has allowed the possibility to identify specific markers and HCC phenotypes as in the case of Keratin 19, considered an invasive progenitor-cell marker.

Furthermore, potential novel tumor markers and molecular signatures for HCC early diagnosis have been identified using modern genomic or proteomic approaches. For example, a 13-gene signature has been described to diagnose HCC lesions with high diagnostic accuracy [14]. In another study, microarray technologies allowed the detection of 120 genes able to differentiate dysplastic nodules from HCC in HBV-patients [15]. Similarly, a three-gene signature (GPC3, LYVE1, and survivin) has been proposed to discriminate between dysplastic nodules and small HCCs (< 2 cm) in HCV-related HCCs [16].

As explained above, many evidences show that HCC diagnosis may require a combination of serum and tissue markers or "molecular signatures." Accordingly, markers such as glypican 3, HSP-70, CD34, CK7 and glutamine synthetase have been included in the new American and European guidelines to improve diagnostic accuracy of small lesions. Furthermore, the European Association for the Study of the Liver (EASL) recommended staining with GPC3, LYVE1, and survivin in addition to detection of progenitor cell features by Keratin19 and EpCAM [9].

References

[1] Walsh KM, Timms P, Campbell S, MacSween RN, Morris AJ. 1999. "Plasma levels of matrix metalloproteinase-2 (MMP-2) and tissue inhibitors of metalloproteinases -1 and -2 (TIMP-1 and TIMP-2) as noninvasive markers of liver disease in chronic hepatitis C: comparison using ROC analysis." *Dig Dis Sci* 44:624-30.

[2] Imbert-Bismut F, Ratziu V, Pieroni L, Charlotte F, Benhamou Y, Poynard T; MULTIVIRC Group. 2001. "Biochemical markers of liver fibrosis in patients with hepatitis C virus infection: a prospective study." *Lancet* 357:1069-75.

[3] Trevisani F, De Notariis S, Rapaccini G, Farinati F, Benvegnù L, Zoli M, Grazi GL, Del PP, Di N, Bernardi M; Italian Liver Cancer Group. 2002. "Semiannual and annual surveillance of cirrhotic patients for

hepatocellular carcinoma: effects on cancer stage and patient survival (Italian Experience)." *Am J Gastroenterol* 97: 734-44.

[4] Bruix J, Boix L, Sala M, Llovet JM. 2004. "Focus on hepatocellular carcinoma." *Cancer Cell.* 5:215-9.

[5] Zhang BH, Yang BH, Tang ZY. 2004. "Randomized controlled trial of screening for hepatocellular carcinoma." *J Cancer Res Clin Oncol* 130:417-22.

[6] Singal A, Volk ML, Waljee A, Salgia R, Higgins P, Rogers MA, Marrero JA. 2009. "Meta-analysis: surveillance with ultrasound for early-stage hepatocellular carcinoma in patients with cirrhosis." *Aliment Pharmacol Ther* 30:37-47. Accessed April 8, 2009. doi: 10.1111/j.1365-2036.2009.04014.

[7] Park MJ, Kim YK, Lee MW, Lee WJ, Kim YS, Kim SH, Choi D, Rhim H. 2012. "Small hepatocellular carcinomas: improved sensitivity by combining gadoxetic acid-enhanced and diffusion-weighted MR imaging patterns." *Radiology* 264:761-70.

[8] Inoue T, Kudo M, Komuta M, Hayaishi S, Ueda T, Takita M, Kitai S, Hatanaka K, Yada N, Hagiwara S, Chung H, Sakurai T, Ueshima K, Sakamoto M, Maenishi O, Hyodo T, Okada M, Kumano S, and Murakami T. 2012. "Assessment of Gd-EOB-DTPA-enhanced MRI for HCC and dysplastic nodules and comparison of detection sensitivity versus MDCT." *J Gastroenterol* 47:1036-47. Accessed April 17, 2012. doi: 10.1007/s00535-012-0571-6.

[9] European Association For The Study Of The Liver, European Organisation For Research And Treatment Of Cancer. 2012. "EASL-EORTC clinical practice guidelines: management of hepatocellular carcinoma." *J Hepatol* 56:908-43.

[10] Roskams T, and Kojiro M. 2010. "Pathology of early hepatocellular carcinoma: conventional and molecular diagnosis." *Semin Liver Dis* 30:17-25. Accessed February 19, 2010. doi: 10.1055/s-0030-1247129.

[11] Taketa K, Endo Y, Sekiya C, Tanikawa K, Koji T, Taga H, Satomura S, Matsuura S, Kawai T, Hirai H. 1993. "A collaborative study for the evaluation of lectin-reactive alpha-fetoproteins in early detection of hepatocellular carcinoma." *Cancer Res* 53:5419-23.

[12] Nomura F, Ishijima M, Horikoshi A, Nakai T, Ohnishi K. 1996. "Determination of serum des-gamma-carboxyprothrombin levels in patients with small-sized hepatocellular carcinoma: comparison of the conventional enzyme immunoassay and two modified methods." *Am J Gastroenterol* 91:1380-3.

[13] Ishii M, Gama H, Chida N, Ueno Y, Shinzawa H, Takagi T, Toyota T, Takahashi T, Kasukawa R. 2000. "Simultaneous measurements of serum alpha-fetoprotein and protein induced by vitamin K absence for detecting hepatocellular carcinoma. South Tohoku District Study Group." *Am J Gastroenterol* 95:1036-40.

[14] Paradis V, Bièche I, Dargère D, Laurendeau I, Laurent C, Bioulac Sage P, Degott C, Belghiti J, Vidaud M, Bedossa P. 2003. "Molecular profiling of hepatocellular carcinomas (HCC) using a large-scale real-time RT-PCR approach: determination of a molecular diagnostic index." *Am J Pathol* 163:733-41.

[15] Nam SW, Park JY, Ramasamy A, Shevade S, Islam A, Long PM, Park CK, Park SE, Kim SY, Lee SH, Park WS, Yoo NJ, Liu ET, Miller LD, Lee JY. 2005. "Molecular changes from dysplastic nodule to hepatocellular carcinoma through gene expression profiling." *Hepatology* 42:809-18.

[16] Llovet JM, Chen Y, Wurmbach E, Roayaie S, Fiel MI, Schwartz M, Thung SN, Khitrov G, Zhang W, Villanueva A, Battiston C, Mazzaferro V, Bruix J, Waxman S, Friedman SL. 2006. "A molecular signature to discriminate dysplastic nodules from early hepatocellular carcinoma in HCV cirrhosis." *Gastroenterology* 131:1758-67.

Chapter 7

Clinical Aspects of HCC: The Prognosis

Evaluation of HCC in an early phase is very important because this allows more effective therapies. However, according to survival rates and patient outcomes reported from studies in "untreated HCCs" - which represent the best representation of HCC natural history - prognosis of this cancer is still largely undefined. For example, a study including 22 eastern cirrhotic patients presenting a tumor 3 cm in diameter reported survival rates of 91, 55 and 13% at 1, 2 and 3 years, respectively [1]. Studies in patients with "advanced unresectable HCC" have been also conducted, reporting survival rates at 1, 2, 3 and 5 years of 54–72, 40–41, 28–38 and 20%, respectively [2-3]. About one-third of patients with advanced HCC presented vascular invasion at 3 years after diagnosis. However, only 22% of patients develop metastasis during this period, more commonly in lungs, local lymphnodes, bone and adrenal glands [2]. The "terminal" stage of disease is characterized by replacement of tumor mass exceeding 50% of liver, vascular invasion and systemic symptoms, with survival ranges from several weeks to a few months. Cancer progression is the most frequent cause of death in HCC patients. The others include liver failure (7–30%), digestive bleeding (7–10%), infections (2%) and pulmonary embolism (1%). Tumor rupture with intraperitoneal bleeding is uncommon in Western countries. The most important factors for prognosis prediction in HCC are hereafter listed. These include tumoral and host factors, whose interaction strongly influence HCC natural history in a not predictable way.

Tumoral Factors Predictive of Prognosis

Tumor size is a significant risk factor associated with vascular invasion, histological grade, decreased disease-free and overall survival. Multiplicity of tumors is also an adverse prognostic factor. Multifocal disease could be the result of intrahepatic metastases from one dominant tumor or multicentric de novo tumors. The presence of microscopic satellite nodules is an indicator of intrahepatic metastasis. To differentiate metastatic tumor nodules from multicentric ones, gene expression profiling has been used in order to evaluate clonality or similar features of multifocal tumors. Furthermore, lymph nodal metastases have a significant negative effect on prognosis, even if hepatic resection with regional lymph node dissection is performed. Another factor to consider is encapsulation. It is well known that well-encapsulated HCCs have a better prognosis than poor encapsulated HCCs or than those with infiltrative growth. However, well encapsulated and nonnecrotic HCCs have a higher tumor pressure gradient associated with venous invasion or intrahepatic metastasis. Poon and collaborators reported that high microvessel density could be a significant predictor of poor disease-free survival after HCC resection [4]. Indeed, patients with multiple tumors, none of them larger than 5 cm, displayed similar prognosis to patients with a single tumor with vascular invasion. Furthermore, the study reported that tumor multiplicity and size did not influence patient outcomes if major vascular invasion was present. This evidence suggests that major vascular invasion can be considered the most important prognostic factor in HCC. In addition, microscopic vascular invasion in histopathological examination is considered the most consistently reported risk factor of postoperative recurrence after resection or liver transplantation. Also, portal vein thrombosis (PVT) is relevant for patient outcomes, as shown in a study where the 5-year survival rate of HCC patients without PVT after surgery was much higher than those with PVT (63.9% vs 40.8%) [5]. Another important factor is inflammation. It has been reported that patients with HCC tumors smaller than 3 cm in diameter with marked inflammatory infiltration showed a significant lower recurrence rate after resection than controls (9.1% vs 47.7%) and higher 5-year survival rate (100% vs 65.1%) presumably due to the antitumoral effect of T lymphocytes [6].

Several authors have better studied the cythological features of tumor in relation with prognosis. For example, cell differentiation is related to faster growth and higher risk of vascular invasion and metastasis and further observations reveal significant differences between hystological subtypes. In particular, trabecular type of HCC is associated with longer volume doubling time. The hepatoblast subtype of HCC, which shares a gene expression pattern with fetal hepatoblasts, has a worse prognosis than the hepatocyte subtype. This subtype may arise from bipotential adult hepatic progenitors cells or from a dedifferentiation process of transformed mature hepatocytes. Considering the heterogeneity of cell-types involved in the transformation process, four prognostic HCC subtypes have been identified, corresponding to different liver cell lineages. Those with the poorest prognosis show a large proportion of $EpCAM^+$ AFP^+ cells (hepatoblast-like) or $EpCAM^-$ AFP^+ cells (HPC-like), whereas those subtypes with $EpCAM^-AFP^-$ cells (mature hepatocyte-like) or $EpCAM^+$ AFP^- cells (cholangiocyte-like) display a more favorable outcome. It has been described that many cancers may contain a subpopulation of self-renewing cells, the so-called *cancer stem cells* (CSCs) that are believed entirely responsible of sustaining the tumor proliferating and differentiating cells. Prominin-1 or CD133, a pentaspan membrane protein, has been proposed as a CSC marker in many different tumors. Using the CD133/1 antibody, it has been shown that CSC represents a very small population (<2%) in primary HCCs. However, continued passages of these cells cause a significant increase in $CD133^+$ cells up to 90%. HCCs with $CD133^+$cells higher than the median number (1.32%) have been correlated with shorter survival, higher recurrence rates, higher tumor grade and higher resistance to conventional therapeutic drugs, such as 5-fluorouracil and doxorubicin [7-8]. As pointed out above, AFP is not very useful for HCC screening because of its low sensitivity and specificity. However, it is extremely useful to evaluate prognosis, therapy response and the possibility of recurrence. Higher AFP levels at diagnosis are related to greater tumor size, bilobar hepatic involvement, portal vein thrombosis and lower survival rate. In fact, the median survival rates of HCC patients with AFP serum levels < 400 IU/mL (6-7 months) are significantly longer than those with AFP levels ≥ 400IU/ mL (3months) [9]. AFP mRNA in peripheral blood might be predictive for early intrahepatic recurrence and metastasis after HCC resection.

As regards the other markers, AFP-L3 is considered a useful indicator of distant metastases and poor prognosis whereas measurement of DCP could be effective in predicting HCC recurrence. Angiogenetic factors represent another category of prognostic determinants that may predict tumor relapse. Several studies have demonstrated a significant correlation between high VEGF expression and poor outcome. Serum and tissue levels of VEGF are correlated with high proliferative index, cellular degree of dedifferentiation, microvascular density, vascular invasion and poor encapsulation. Moreover, enhanced expression of HIF-1A was found in tumors with poor prognosis and high recurrence rate after resection [10-11].

Markers of proliferation (i.e., PCNA, Ki67, cyclins and cyclin-dependent kinases) and telomerase activity have also been employed as predictive factors of HCC relapse after resection. Independent reports have observed a relation between chromosomal losses or gains and poor prognosis in HCC. For example, chromosome losses on 9p and 6q are specifically associated with a poor outcome [12]. Chromosomal instability and p53 mutations have been associated to HBV infection and poor differentiation in HCC. Mutation of p53 gene has also been related to a decreased survival whereas the reduced expression of p27 and other "cell-cycle inhibitors" have been found as an independent predictor of poor prognosis [10]. Other reports have described more frequent β-catenin mutations in well-differentiated HCCs. DNA aneuploidy seems to be related to increased risk of postoperative HCC recurrence [13]. HCC progression and poor outcome have been related with enhanced activity of "apoptosis inhibitors," as BCL-xL, survivin, PTMA and SET [10-11]. With regard to cell adhesion molecules, the reduced expression of E-caderin predicts a poor prognosis. Matrix metalloproteinases and the plasminogen activator system are well known to be involved in metastatic behavior [10]. Hormonal and growth factors alterations have also been related to prognosis. For example, activating mutations of estrogen receptors correlate with poor outcome in HCC [3] and growth-promoting factors such as c-myc, ras and HGF or c-met and the ErbB receptor family may be useful prognostic molecular markers in HCC [10]. In addition, overexpression of leptin receptors may predict a better survival [10] as well as elevated levels of placenta growth factor may be indicators of early HCC recurrence after resection [14].

In order to get a better prognostic risk stratification of HCC patients, several scoring systems have been proposed. For example, a scoring system predicting recurrence and survival after HCC resection has been reported by el-Assal and collegues [15]. This scoring consists of six variables including invasion of portal vein, intrahepatic dissemination, hepatic vein invasion, serosal invasion, absence of tumor capsule or capsule invasion. According to this system, HCCs may be divided into three groups namely low HCC invasiveness (A: 0-1 scores), middle HCC invasiveness (B: 2-4 scores) and high HCC invasiveness (C: 5-11 scores). Recently, a great interest has focused in the characterization of gene expression profile trough cDNA microarray tecniques to better predicte prognosis and HCC recurrence, identifying different HCC survival subclasses. According to the study by Lee and collaborators, the low survival subclass included tumors with a strong expression of cell proliferation and antiapoptosis genes. In addition, this low survival subclass of HCCs displays higher expression of HIF-1A and genes involved in ubiquitination (probably involved in selective degradation of cellcycle inhibitors) and enhanced expression of histone variants involved in response to chromosome breaks and genomic instability [11]. Gene expression profiling could also be useful to identify HCC subsets having a profile indicating an origin from HPCs, which is known to correlate to worse prognosis. Enumeration of CK19-positive cells in HCC could identify a subset of patients who have a shorter time to recurrence. Furthermore, the study of gene expression profiling has been proposed to differentiate metastatic tumor nodules (intrahepatic metastases) from multicentric occurring nodules by evaluating multifocal tumors clonality. Several studies proposed specific molecular signatures to predict recurrence and patient outcomes in surgically resected HCC. A PCR wide-analysis using an array of 3072 genes carried out by Kurokawa and coworkers in 100 HCC patients undergoing liver resection revealed that a 20 gene-molecular signature was an independent indicator for recurrence [16]. In another study, molecular analysis of 63 selected genes predicted patient response to therapy [17]. Villanueva and collegues, analyzing 22 gene signatures, identified "the G3-proliferation signature" from tumor and "the poor-survival signature" from adjacent nontumoral tissue as independent predictors of HCC recurrence [18]. Furthermore, in another study, the same authors proposed a gene expression score including five genes (TAF9, RAMP3, HN1, KRT19 and RAN) to predict survival and early HCC recurrence after resection [19].

Host Factors Predictive of Prognosis

In addition to tumor factors, host factors may also influence HCC prognosis. Patient general conditions including age, sex, co-existing hepatitis, fibrosis, and liver function have a prognostic value among these factors. Clinical observations suggest that female HCC patients have more frequently well-encapsulated and less invasive tumor with lower recurrent rate and better prognosis than male HCC patients. These might be due to the different expression of estrogen and androgen receptors in HCC. Indeed, ER positive HCCs have less malignant biologic behavior and a better prognosis than ER negative HCCs. The presence of variant ER transcripts in inoperable HCCs shows spontaneous survival significantly worse than that of patients with wild-type ER [3]. Also, age has a relevant prognostic value. Younger HCC patients (< 35 years) tend to have more aggressive tumor behavior than elderly, with faster growing, higher invasive and metastatic potential and higher recurrence rate. The inflammatory activity and the hepatic reserve have been considered two important risk factors for recurrence in these patients. It is well known that the postoperative overall and disease-free survival rates of patients without viral infection are better than HCC patients with HBV infection or with HBV-HCV co-infection. HBsAg seronegative patients show a greater postoperative long-term survival rate than HBsAg seropositive patients. Furthermore, a high viral load is an independent risk factor for recurrence as evidenced in a study where HCC patients with middle hepatitis histological activity (hepatitis activity index – HAI – score = 6-9) in non-tumoral hepatic tissue had a higher intrahepatic recurrent rate [20]. Etiology of cirrhosis is determinant in HCC patient outcomes. Patients with alcoholic liver disease or HCV infection usually experience poorer outcomes than HBV patients undergoing resection [21] and this may be partly explained by considering the possibility of some HBV-associated HCCs to bypass the cirrhotic state. However, patients with HCV- or alcohol-related HCCs experience better outcomes with sorafenib [22]. Another independent prognostic factor is the functional reserve of the remnant cirrhotic liver. In particular, hepatic dysfunction immediately after hepatectomy is an important risk factor for early intrahepatic recurrence. Markers of hepatic function including albumin, prothrombin time, alanine transaminase, gamma-glutamyl transpeptidase and the 15-minute indocyanine green retention rate have an important predictive value for disease-free survival in HCC patients. However, the Child-Pugh score still remains the gold standard as predictor of prognosis in HCC patients. As for other tumors, HCC natural history is influenced by the host immune response. For example, immunosuppression in HIV^+ HCC patients is associated to a worse prognosis. Moreover, the density of lymphocyte infiltration in the nodule (a surrogate marker of the antitumoral immune response) and the activation of the host NK cells are inversely correlated with malignant potential and the risk of recurrence after resection. Finally, the relative predominance of negative immune modulator CD4þ/CD25þ lymphocytes in the blood or peritumoral tissue could be associated with HCC development and progression.

Recent studies indicate that prognosis of recurrent HCC after resection is dependent on the time of recurrence. In particular, in one study, prognosis for patients with early (≤ 1 year) recurrence was worse than that of patients with late (> 1 year) recurrence [23]. Preoperative tumor rupture, serum albumin level, initial TNM staging and venous invasion were independent risk factors for early recurrence, whereas cirrhosis and serum bilirubin levels were significant risk factors for late recurrence.

Table 3. Tumoral/Host factors for predicting prognosis in patients with HCC. HCC patient outcomes can be influenced by several tumoral factors including tumor size and multiplicity, microscopic satellite nodules, lymph nodal metastases, encapsulation, microvessel density, vascular invasion, PVT, cell differentiation, inflammatory cell infiltration, hystological subtype, tumoral markers, genetic and epigenetic factors. Not less important in prognosis prediction are host factors as age, sex, liver functional reserve, HAI, etiology of cirrhosis, host immune response and time of recurrence

Tumoral factors	Host factors
Tumor size	Age
Multiplicity of tumors	Sex
Microscopic satellite nodules	Liver functional reserve /Child Pugh score
Lymph nodal metastases	Hepatitis activity index (HAI)
Encapsulation	Etiology of cirrhosis
Microvessel density	Host immune response
Vascular invasion	Time of recurrence
PVT (portal vein trombosis)	
Cell differentiation	
Inflammatory cell infiltration	
Hystological Subtype - prevalence of: $EpCAM^{+}AFP^{+}$ (hepatoblast-like cells) $EpCAM^{-}AFP^{+}$ (HPC-like cells) CD133+ (CSC cells)	
Tumoral markers	
Chromosome abnormalities	
Gene signature	
Expression of: -markers of proliferation/angiogenesis -cell cycle/apoptosis inhibitors -cell adhesion molecules -matrix metalloproteinases -hormonal and growth factors	

Clinical Staging

It is well known that clinical stage is one of the most important determinants of prognosis in patients with HCC. The TNM system evaluates tumor features (T), the presence or absence of lymph nodes involvement (N) and distant metastasis (M). Other informations are histologic grade (G) and fibrosis score (F) based on the Ishak classification. A new T staging system has been proposed to better predict the outcome of patients after curative liver resection. In this new system, T1 is defined as no vascular invasion, small size (≤ 5cm), and solitary tumor; T2 as the presence of one of the following factors: size greater than 5 cm, vascular invasion, or multiple tumors; T3 as the presence of two of the above three factors; and T4 as the presence of all three factors. Portal vein invasion (Vp) and intrahepatic metastasis (IM) reflect the invasive properties of HCC.

The MELD score is a logarithmic score that includes PT INR (prothrombin time international normalized ratio), serum creatinine, total serum bilirubin and the etiology of cirrhosis. It is widely used in the field of liver transplantation to prioritize donor liver allocation by prediction of short-term mortality. However, it fails to correctly classify a portion of patients with advanced cirrhosis.

The Child Pugh (CP) score is the most used grading system for liver function. CP A includes patients with normal liver function and a 100% 12-month survival without HCC or without any treatment. Patients classified as CP C have poor liver function and need transplantation, considering that, without transplant, their survival is usually 40% at 12 months, with or without HCC. Patients classified as CP B score are an intermediate heterogeneous group with a 60% 12-month survival without HCC or without any treatment. The Child-Turcotte-Pug (CTP) score has several limits that include inter-laboratory variations, daily parameters fluctuations and the subjective evaluation of the clinical grading of encephalopathy and ascites. It has also been proposed an IGF-modified CTP staging that includes serum insulin-like growth factor-1 (IGF-1) as a surrogate for hepatic function since its production is reduced in cirrhosis [24].

The CTP score has been included into scoring systems such as Barcelona Clinic Liver Cancer (BCLC), Cancer of the Liver Italian Program (CLIP) and Japan Integrated Staging (JIS). The CLIP score and the BCLC system are both commonly used in Europe, whereas the JIS score is widely used in Japan and other Asian regions, but it has not been validated in a Western population.

The BCLC system gives important indications for therapy. In fact, patients are allocated to a specific treatment plan based on tumor burden, size and number of nodules, presence of satellites or extrahepatic spread, liver function (Child-Pugh classification) and symptoms (i.e. ECOG Performance status test). This designates HCC as 1 of the 5 stages: the very early stage (stage 0) and early stage (stage A) tumors amenable to potentially curative treatment (resection or local ablation or liver transplantation); intermediate (stage B) tumors treated by transarterial chemoembolization (TACE); advanced (stage C) tumors treated with sorafenib and terminal (stage D) tumors treated with supportive care. However, BCLC stage B includes a heterogeneous population of HCCs with a large variety of tumor size (ranging from small to near complete replacement of the liver) and with different liver function (ranging from preserved to compromised performance status). Therefore, this large variability allows some BCLC stage B patients to be treated following BCLC stage C algorithms.

The CLIP score (range 0-5) includes Child-Pugh stage, tumor morphology, AFP level and the presence or absence of portal vein thrombosis.

The JIS score might be superior in survival prediction compared to CLIP, especially in patients with early stage disease. This score incorporates the modification of the Liver Cancer Study Group of Japan (LCSGJ) classification of the TNM system and the Child-Pugh score.

Other prognostic scoring systems are the Okuda system, the Chinese University Prognostic Index (CUPI) and the French scoring system. The Okuda system includes tumor burden, the presence or absence of ascites, serum albumin and bilirubin levels. The CUPI score has been proposed to predict survival in Asian patients with advanced HCC. However, in western populations, with a greater HCV prevalence, the CUPI score has not been validated. The parameters included are TNM stage, asymptomatic disease on presentation, ascites, AFP, serum total bilirubin and alkaline phosphatase. The French scoring system includes performance status by Karnofsky score, serum bilirubin, serum alkaline phosphatase, AFP, and presence or absence of portal obstruction by ultrasonography. The limit could be the alterations of the sensitivity for portal obstruction and, to date, this system has not improved prognostic stratification of patients comparing to other scores.

As mentioned in the above paragraph, the heterogeneous nature of HCC has made difficult to implement an accepted universal staging system and each of the newly proposed prognostical systems has several limitations. None of these algorithms, for example, include tumor location and proximity to major vessels, anatomical and biological variables of HCC.

References

[1] Ebara M, Ohto M, Shinagawa T, Sugiura N, Kimura K, Matsutani S, Morita M, Saisho H, Tsuchiya Y, Okuda K. 1986. "Natural history of minute hepatocellular carcinoma smaller than three centimeters complicating cirrhosis. A study in 22 patients." *Gastroenterology* 90: 289-98.

[2] Llovet JM, Bustamante J, Castells A, Vilana R, Ayuso Mdel C, Sala M, Brú C, Rodés J, Bruix J. 1999. "Natural history of untreated nonsurgical hepatocellular carcinoma: rationale for the design and evaluation of therapeutic trials." *Hepatology* 29:62-7.

[3] Villa E, Moles A, Ferretti I, Buttafoco P, Grottola A, Del Buono M, De Santis M, Manenti F. 2000. "Natural history of inoperable hepatocellular carcinoma: estrogen receptors' status in the tumor is the strongest prognostic factor for survival." *Hepatology* 32:233-8.

[4] Poon RT, Ng IO, Lau C, Yu WC, Yang ZF, Fan ST, Wong J. 2002. "Tumor microvessel density as a predictor of recurrence after resection of hepatocellular carcinoma: a prospective study." *J Clin Oncol* 20: 1775-85.

[5] Qin LX, Tang ZY. 2002. "The prognostic significance of clinical and patho-logical features in hepatocellular carcinoma." *World J Gastroenterol* 8: 193-9.

[6] Wada Y, Nakashima O, Kutami R, Yamamoto O, Kojiro M. 1998. "Clinicopathological study on hepatocellular carcinoma with lymphocytic infiltration." *Hepatology* 27:407-14.

[7] Song W, Li H, Tao K, Li R, Song Z, Zhao Q, Zhang F, and Dou K. 2008. "Expression and clinical significance of the stem cell marker CD133 in hepatocellular carcinoma." *Int J Clin Pract* 62:1212-8. Accessed May 8, 2008. doi: 10.1111/j.1742-1241.2008.01777.x.

[8] Ma S, Lee TK, Zheng BJ, Chan KW, Guan XY. 2008. "CD133+ HCC cancer stem cells confer chemoresistance by preferential expression of the Akt/PKB survival pathway." *Oncogene* 27:1749-58.

[9] Tangkijvanich P, Anukulkarnkusol N, Suwangool P, Lertmaharit S, Hanvivatvong O, Kullavanijaya P, Poovorawan Y. 2000. "Clinical characteristics and prognosis of hepatocellular carcinoma: analysis based on serum alpha-fetoprotein levels." *J Clin Gastroenterol* 31:302-8.

[10] Mann CD, Neal CP, Garcea G, Manson MM, Dennison AR, Berry DP. 2007. "Prognostic molecular markers in hepatocellular carcinoma: a systematic review." *Eur J Cancer* 43:979-92.

[11] Lee JS, Chu IS, Heo J, Calvisi DF, Sun Z, Roskams T, Durnez A, Demetris AJ, Thorgeirsson SS. 2004. "Classification and prediction of survival in hepatocellular carcinoma by gene expression profiling." *Hepatology* 40:667-76.

[12] Laurent-Puig P, Legoix P, Bluteau O, Belghiti J, Franco D, Binot F, Monges G, Thomas G, Bioulac-Sage P, Zucman-Rossi J. 2001. "Genetic alterations associated with hepatocellular carcinomas define distinct pathways of hepatocarcinogenesis." *Gastroenterology* 120:1763-73.

[13] Chiu JH, Kao HL, Wu LH, Chang HM, Lui WY. 1992. "Prediction of relapse or survival after resection in human hepatomas by DNA flow cytometry." *J Clin Invest* 89:539-45.

[14] Ho MC, Chen CN, Lee H, Hsieh FJ, Shun CT, Chang CL, Lai YT, Lee PH. 2007. "Placenta growth factor not vascular endothelial growth factor A or C can predict the early recurrence after radical resection of hepatocellular carcinoma." *Cancer Lett* 250:237-49.

[15] el-Assal ON, Yamanoi A, Soda Y, Yamaguchi M, Yu L, Nagasue N. 1997. "Proposal of invasiveness score to predict recurrence and survival after curative hepatic resection for hepatocellular carcinoma." *Surgery* 122:571-7.

[16] Kurokawa Y, Matoba R, Takemasa I, Nagano H, Dono K, Nakamori S, Umeshita K, Sakon M, Ueno N, Oba S, Ishii S, Kato K, Monden M. 2004. "Molecular-based prediction of early recurrence in hepatocellular carcinoma." *J Hepatol* 41:284-91.

[17] Kurokawa Y, Matoba R, Nagano H, Sakon M, Takemasa I, Nakamori S, Dono K, Umeshita K, Ueno N, Ishii S, Kato K, Monden M. 2004. "Molecular prediction of response to 5-fluorouracil and interferon-alpha combination chemotherapy in advanced hepatocellular carcinoma." *Clin Cancer Res* 10:6029-38.

[18] Villanueva A, Hoshida Y, Battiston C, Tovar V, Sia D, Alsinet C, Cornella H, Liberzon A, Kobayashi M, Kumada H, Thung SN, Bruix J, Newell P, April C, Fan JB, Roayaie S, Mazzaferro V, Schwartz ME, and Llovet JM. 2011. "Combining clinical, pathology, and gene expression data to predict recurrence of hepatocellular carcinoma." *Gastroenterology* 140:1501-12.e2. Accessed February 12, 2011. doi: 10.1053/j.gastro.2011.02.006.

[19] Nault JC, De Reyniès A, Villanueva A, Calderaro J, Rebouissou S, Couchy G, Decaens T, Franco D, Imbeaud S, Rousseau F, Azoulay D, Saric J, Blanc JF,Balabaud C, Bioulac-Sage P, Laurent A, Laurent-Puig P, Llovet JM, and Zucman-Rossi J. 2013. "A hepatocellular carcinoma 5-gene score associated with survival of patients after liver resection." *Gastroenterology* 145:176-87. Accessed April 6, 2013. doi: 10.1053/ j.gastro.2013.03.051.

[20] Ueno S, Tanabe G, Yoshida A, Yoshidome S, Takao S, Aikou T. 1999. "Postoperative prediction of and strategy for metastatic recurrent hepatocellular carcinoma according to histologic activity of hepatitis." *Cancer* 86:248-54.

[21] Huang YH, Wu JC, Chen CH, Chang TT, Lee PC, Chau GY, Lui WY, Chang FY, Lee SD. 2005. "Comparison of recurrence after hepatic resection in patients with hepatitis B vs. hepatitis C-related small hepatocellular carcinoma in hepatitis B virus endemic area." *Liver Int* 25:236-41.

[22] Bruix J, Raoul JL, Sherman M, Mazzaferro V, Bolondi L, Craxi A, Galle PR, Santoro A, Beaugrand M, Sangiovanni A, Porta C, Gerken G, Marrero JA, Nadel A,Shan M, Moscovici M, Voliotis D, and Llovet JM. 2012. "Efficacy and safety of sorafenib in patients with advanced hepatocellular carcinoma: subanalyses of a phase III trial." *J Hepatol* 57:821-9. Accessed June 19, 2012. doi: 10.1016/j.jhep.2012.06.014.

[23] Poon RT, Fan ST, Ng IO, Lo CM, Liu CL, Wong J. 2000. "Different risk factors and prognosis for early and late intrahepatic recurrence after resection of hepatocellular carcinoma." *Cancer* 89:500-7.

[24] Kaseb AO, Morris JS, Hassan MM, Siddiqui AM, Lin E, Xiao L, Abdalla EK, Vauthey JN, Aloia TA, Krishnan S, and Abbruzzese JL. 2011. "Clinical and prognostic implications of plasma insulin-like growth factor-1 and vascular endothelial growth factor in patients with hepatocellular carcinoma." *J Clin Oncol* 29:3892-9. Accessed September 12, 2011. doi: 10.1200/JCO.2011.36.0636.

Chapter 8

Clinical Aspects of HCC: The Prevention

Neonatal vaccination against HBV is already showing a significant decrease in both HBV and HCC incidence among children and adolescents in endemic areas. The elimination of HCV-contaminated blood in European and Asian blood banks is expected to contribute to a great decrease in HCV infection. Prevention of *Aspergillus* from growing, by storing grains in refrigerated silos, is likely the most effective preventive measure in areas where this mold is considered the most relevant risk factor for HCC. Intervention in changing life style, in particular alcohol consumption, is important but the effects could be greater when undertaken at younger age or at earlier phases of the hepatitis. As deduced from the knowledge of cancer pathobiology, effective antiviral therapies have a crucial role in HCC prevention. Treatment with lamivudine may prevent HCC development in chronic hepatitis B [1]. However, long-term suppression of HBV replication is mandatory to continuously reduce HCC incidence. To achieve this goal, two problems should be overcome. First, the development of resistant strains during therapy. Second, the progression of hepatitis and the persistence of (ccc) HBV DNA as a consequence of drug suspension. Recent studies revealed that adefovir, dipivoxil and entecavir show lower emergence rates of resistant viral strains. Accordingly, the combination of these anti-viral drugs has been proposed. Also, combination therapy with peginterferon-alpha 2b and ribavirin for 24 (serotype 2) to 48 (genotypes 1a and 1b) weeks is recommended to reduce the incidence of HCC in HCV patients. More recently, new direct-acting antivirals (DAAs) for the treatment of chronic hepatitis C have revolutionized the current status of HCV treatment and they are intended for having a huge impact on the prevention of HCC. Finally, some studies have demonstrated the role of certain vitamins in the prevention of HCC. In particular, vitamin K2 (menaquinone) may play a role in HCC prevention in women with viral cirrhosis probably through the control of cell growth. Synthetic analogues of vitamin A with agonistic activity for the nuclear retinoid receptors such as acyclic retinoids or polyprenoic acid have also been studied in HCC prevention. Considering that acyclic retinoids and interferon would have both a cancer preventive action, although by different mechanisms, and synergistic effects in inducing apoptosis in HCC cells, a combination therapy has been proposed [2].

References

[1] Matsumoto A, Tanaka E, Rokuhara A, Kiyosawa K, Kumada H, Omata M, Okita K, Hayashi N, Okanoue T, Iino S, Tanikawa K, Inuyama Hepatitis Study Group. 2005. "Efficacy of lamivudine for preventing hepatocellular carcinoma in chronic hepatitis B: a multicenter retrospective study of 2795 patients." *Hepatol Res* 32:173-84.

[2] Obora A, Shiratori Y, Okuno M, Adachi S, Takano Y, Matsushima-Nishiwaki R, Yasuda I, Yamada Y, Akita K, Sano T, Shimada J, Kojima S, Okano Y, Friedman SL, Moriwaki H. 2002. "Synergistic induction of apoptosis by acyclic retinoid and interferon-beta in human hepatocellular carcinoma cells." *Hepatology* 36:1115-24.

Chapter 9

Clinical Aspects of HCC: The Therapy

Main Therapies

Several factors influence the therapeutic choice in patients with HCC, such as stadiation, tumor biology and liver dysfunction degree. Currently, numerous therapeutic choices are available for HCC. These include local ablative therapies such as cryosurgery, radiofrequency ablation, microwave ablation or percutaneous ethanol injection, hepatic artery transcatheter treatments, transarterial chemotherapy and radiotherapy, transarterial embolization and chemoembolization, transarterial drug-eluting beads, external beam radiation or surgery (i.e. resection, liver transplantation) and systemic therapies (i.e. sorafenib, chemotherapy, immunotherapy, hormonal therapy) or supportive therapies.

Surgical resection is the treatment of choice for patients in early stage (BCLC 0-1) with good performance status and preserved liver function. A recent meta-analysis showed that the overall survival after resection has been improved over the years with an expected 5-year survival of 60% [1]. However, recurrence rate exceeds 50% in 2 years. As regards the risk of procedure, a low perioperative mortality rate (3%) with a low rate of intraoperative blood transfusion (<10%) has been reported [2] The recent advances in laparoscopic liver resection have significantly improved patient outcomes compared with the open approach obtaining similar long-term survival, with reported reduced operative blood loss and hospital lenght of stay

[3]. The most important factor influencing perioperative mortality and long-term survival after hepatectomy is the underlying hepatic function according to the Child Pugh Score. Other factors to be considered are the presence and the severity of portal hypertension evaluated by the 15-minute indocyanine green retention rate, the presence of splenomegaly, the hepatic venous pressure gradient measurement and the serum platelet count. An important consideration about the preoperative planning is the assessment of postoperative future liver remnant (FLR) volume for predicting the postresection liver function. The total liver volume and FLR volume are directly measured on CT or MRI scans. Calculation of the FLR volume is an important parameter to select patients with inadequate reserve who may benefit from preoperative liver hypertrophy-procedures, as for patients candidate to the portal vein embolization (PVE). This procedure consists in embolizing the portal vein that provides flow to the liver portion wherein the tumor is present, with consequent hypertrophy of the contralateral liver. In a large meta-analysis, Abulkhir et al. reported that PVE increased FLR volume from 8% to 27% with a morbidity rate of 2.2% and no mortality [4]. The liver partition with portal vein ligation is another proposed hypertrophy-inducing strategy for staging hepatectomy (ALPPS) effective in liver volume increasing (median rate of 74% in about 9 days) but encumbered by a procedure-related morbidity rate of 68% and mortality rate of 12% [5]. According to the NCCN and the EASL-EORTC guidelines, hepatectomy is the most accreditated therapy for patients with early stage HCC (one tumor ≤5 cm or ≤3 tumors, each ≤3 cm in size, without macroscopic vascular invasion) and preserved liver function (Child-Pugh A without portal hypertension). An additional NCCN recommendation is that the postoperative FLR volume should be at least 30-40% in patients with Child-Pugh A cirrhosis and 20% in absence of cirrhosis. None of these guidelines have included in its recommendations the actual FLR hypertrophy approaches discussed above. However, PVE is widely used and could be considered as standard of care in case of insufficient FLR volume. Considering that the proportion of Asian patients presenting with resectable HCC is very low (10-15%), half that patients in USA and Europe, likely due to the higher prevalence of HBV and HCV with the consequent host hepatic reserve impairment, more liberal criteria are considered by the AOS. In fact, patients with solitary tumors or with multifocal tumors (if resection is technically feasible) with preserved liver function, without extrahepatic metastases and gross vascular invasion are candidated for surgical resection. The recent advancements in surgery (i.e. intraoperative projection of CT

images using ultrasound to help in locating intrahepatic tumors) could overcome these limits in future.

Percutaneous treatments, including percutaneous radiofrequency ablation (RFA) or percutaneous ethanol injection (PEI) are recommended for small non-surgical HCCs.

RFA is a good alternative treatment for patients with early HCCs (lesions ≤ 3 cm), not eligible for surgical resection with well-preserved liver function. However, novel probes have also been proposed for single lesions with larger size (up to 5 cm).

PEI allows complete response in about 70% of patients with solitary tumors (< 3 cm) and nearly in 100% of patients with tumor size less than 2 cm. This tecnique is also indicated for patients that cannot be treated by RFA because of the tumor location.

Both ablative therapies and resection have certain limitations. The main limitations are the severity of cirrhosis and the topology of the tumor within the liver. Adjacent HCCs to a major hepatic blood vessel or bile duct have more chances to cause liver damage.

Hepatic Artery Infusion (HAI) or Hepatic Artery Chemoembolization (TACE)

This therapeutic option consists in injecting into hepatic artery high doses of chemotherapy selectively in HCC nodules minimizing the exposure of liver to drug toxicities and the amount of chemotherapy drugs that reaches the systemic circulation. However, the cirrhotic liver is only partially protected because of hepatic arterial blood shunting. Therefore, TACE significantly increases the local concentration of the drug and the anti-tumoral efficacy exploiting the different vascular supply of HCC, compared to the liver, as mentioned above. It causes obstruction of hepatic artery with consequent extensive necrosis in large vascularized HCCs. Embolization agents (i.e. gelatin) are administered by the intra-arterial route with anti-tumoral drugs such as doxorubicin, mitomycin or cisplatin mixed with lipiodol (chemoembolization). Partial responses have been reported in 15% to 55% of patients with a significant delay in tumor progression and vascular invasion [6]. The crucial point of this procedure is a correct selection of patients as candidates for chemo-embolization. Chemoembolization is not considered as the first-line therapy in early stage, but it is recommended in patients with asymptomatic multinodular tumors or extensive HCCs with preserved liver function, not eligible for radical treatments and in absence of vascular invasion or extrahepatic spread (BCLC stage B). On the contrary, liver failure (CTP's B-C) contraindicates this therapeutical choise, since the ischemic insult may cause severe adverse events. It is also contraindicated in the presence of complete PVT and needs great caution if there is evidence of the major branch PVT.

Radioembolization is a locoregional therapy that uses radioactive spheres (20–30 microns diameter) that carry radioactivity from the beta particle-emitting isotope 90Yttrium. Both Thera-Sphere and SIR-Spheres use 90Yttrium labeled spheres. However, they work differently. In fact, while TheraSphere is a pure radiation treatment using much higher doses of radiation, SIR-Spheres have lower radiation dosage but a higher number of spheres per dose, which exert a TACE-like effect. These products have obtained an approval by the FDA as a humanitarian device exemption (HDE). In Japan, it is avalaible another radioisotope, ^{131}I-Lipiodol, showing a minor toxicities and improvement in recurrence free survival after surgical resection. However, no completed randomized trials have marked a gold standard for this therapeutic approach.

Unlike TACE, radioactive spheres can be used for the treatment of HCC confined to the liver also in presence of PVT. Authors showed responses in 35–50% of patients using TACE or radioembolization, with reported average survival of 12-18 months for these unresectable HCCs, according to liver function [7].

External beam radiotherapy, usually, is not employed, considering its hepato-toxicity. It is indicated for treatment of main stem or main branch PVT. However, new technical approaches using more finely focused radiation beams (i.e., modulation of intensity of radiation therapy, stereotactic body radiation) seem to be more promising. A novel therapeutic approach is proton beam therapy that needs to be validated.

Liver transplantation is another curative option that is, when applicable, the only therapeutic option able to cure both HCC and cirrhosis at the same time. Since 1996, the Milan criteria have become the standard tool to individuate patients with HCC elegible to transplantation. The NCCN and EASL-EORTC guidelines, according to the Milan criteria, recommend that only patients who have solitary tumors (less than 5 cm in size) or patients with multifocal disease (no more than 3 nodules each less than 3 cm in size) not eligible for surgical resection should be directed to liver transplantation. Following these criteria the expected four-year overall survival rate is 85% and the recurrence-free survival is 93%. For patients whose tumor cannot be resected or ablated or do not fit within the transplant criteria, reductive treatments such as TACE can be used to decrease tumor size in order to reconsider RFA, surgical resection, or liver transplantation. Furhermore, the

AOS recommend that the Milan criteria can be cautiously expanded for selected cohorts of patients.

A persistent problem is the HCC growth-rate during the waiting period for a donor liver. If tumors are larger than those expected by Milan criteria, the patient is no longer elegible to liver transplantation. This means that patients need to have regular check-up, three-monthly scans and AFP measurements, while on the liver transplant waiting list. TACE, radioembolization, and sorafenib are treatment options for patients awaiting liver transplantation ("bridging therapies"). Although these are treatments commonly carried out to prevent disease progression or to downstaging to reach the Milan criteria for transplantation, they are not formally recommended. Some patients have HCC recurrence after liver transplantation. If the tumor recurrence is confined to the liver, then TACE can be considered. If it is outside the liver monotherapy with sorafenib could be considered. To reduce the recurrence rate after transplantation, aggressive post-operative antiviral therapies are highly recommended, considering the frequent hepatitis recurrence in the transplanted liver. Furhermore, the introduction of cyclosporine as immunosuppression therapy after liver transplantation in the early 1980s has increased patient survival at 1 year from below 20% to over 50%. Actually, survival rates after liver transplantation exceed 85% at 1 year and 70% at 5 years. Considering the frequent relevant complications during liver transplantation, a correct management of patients in perioperative period is very important. The most described complication is certainly the postreperfusion syndrome, characterized by marked hemodynamic alterations that follow revascularization of the liver graft. Another crucial aspect to underline is that guidelines for transplantation in HCC patients cannot be standardized globally considering the differences in regional organ availability and transplantation waiting time.

The presence of metastasis and portal vein thrombosis usually exclude any surgery or regional therapy. Hence, patients with advanced tumors (BCLC stage C and D) showing vascular involvement, extrahepatic spread or physical impairment are assessed for new anti-tumoral agents including *sorafenib*. Sorafenib is a multikinase inhibitor with inhibiting activity against RAS, VEGFR, and PDGFR adopted in clinical guidelines as standard of care for patients with advanced and disseminated HCC. The main indications for sorafenib therapy are i) failure of TACE or radioembolization, ii) cases in which TACE or radioembolization are unsafe iii) metastatic HCCs. Sorafenib is also indicated as "bridging therapy" to liver transplantation in association with TACE or radioembolization. Finally, sorafenib has been proposed as adjuvant therapy to prevent recurrences after tumor resection or ablation. In a comparative study, investigators showed that the median overall survival was 10.7 versus 7.9 months when patients were given sorafenib (400 mg twice daily) or placebo, respectively [8]. Sorafenib was shown to cause a significant decrease in the tumor vascularity on radiology scans, a hallmark of tumor cell viability. However, it was reported a minimal tumor shrinkage (2% partial responses). Consequently tumors were still mostly present with possibility to regrowth. Other limits of sorafenib therapy are represented by the known side effects, such as profound tiredness and weakness (30% of patients) and diarrhea, with consequent discontinuation or cessation of therapy or doses reduction. Another side effect is represented by the *hand–foot syndrome* (in about 10% of patients), which is characterized by redness, swelling, and painful blisters on the palms of the hands and the soles of the feet. Several recent trials have proposed different combination therapies with sorafenib, including sorafenib with other newer kinase inhibitors or sorafenib plus TACE or sorafenib plus radioembolization.

Table 4. Indications and main treatment options for HCC. Surgical resection, percutaneous treatments (RFA, PEI), TACE, radioembolization, external beam radiotherapy, liver transplantation, sorafenib and palliative care represent the actual main standard therapies for HCC patients

Surgical resection	early stage good performance status preserved hepatic function
Percutaneous treatments (RFA, PEI)	small non-surgical HCCs
TACE	asymptomatic multinodular tumors/extensive HCCs preserved liver function not eligible for radical treatments no vascular invasion/extrahepatic spread "bridging therapy" to transplantation
Radioembolization	HCC confined to the liver also in presence of PVT "bridging therapy" to transplantation
External beam radiotherapy	main stem or main branch PVT
Liver transplantation	tumor number ≤ 3, all with size ≤3 cm single tumor or lesion ≤ 5 cm
Sorafenib	advanced and disseminated HCCs after failure of TACE/radioembolization or if unsafe "bridging therapy" to transplantation
Palliative Care	terminal stage (BCLC stage D, Child-Pugh C)

Patients at a terminal stage (BCLC stage D), especially those with a Child-Pugh C, frank liver failure or with obstructive jaundice caused by portal vein thrombosis that are not amenable to the above therapies, need symptomatic or *palliative care* only.

Response to Therapy

The measurement of tumor size and number are significant means to quantify therapy-response. Several accepted response classification schemes have been used, including schemes from the World Health Organization (WHO), response evaluation criteria in solid tumors (RECIST) and recently modified RECIST (mRECIST), the latter particularly useful for HCC. Assessments have included i) complete response/disappearance of tumor; ii) partial response/shrinkage of tumor; iii) stable disease; iv) progressive disease/growth in tumor size or number. Furthermore, a valutation of tumor vascularity on CT or MRI scan could be considered as a measure of decreased tumor viability or increased necrosis. For HCC patients with elevated circulating AFP levels, a consistent reduction of this marker may indicate response to therapy. As described above, several authors have tried to figure out a possible link between specific gene mutations or signatures with HCC recurrence rate after surgery though without clear results. What is well clear is that after surgery two types of HCC recurrence can occur. The early recurrence (<12 months), which may origin from growth of microscopic residual HCC, and the late recurrence, probably generated from new HCCs formed in the cirrhotic pre-malignant nodules. Neo-adjuvant (before resection) and adjuvant (after resection) chemotherapies have been proposed to reduce HCC recurrence incidence.

Adjuvant Therapies

Postoperative adjuvant therapies with TACE, IFN-α, HACE or autologous transplant with recombinant interleukin-2-activated lymphocytes might reduce the three-year recurrent rate after liver resection. In particular, postoperative IFN-alpha therapy has been reported to decrease recurrence after resection of HCV-related HCC [9]. In patients with interferon-resistant HCV, therapy based on glycyrrhizin injection significantly decreased HCC incidence [10].

TACE is particularly useful in treating the postoperative residual tumor, but it could increase the risk of metastatic dissemination. Another proposed adjuvant therapy is that with acyclic retinoid. A study shows that oral administration of retinoid for 48 weeks prevented the formation of a second HCC after radical treatments, with consequent survival improvement [11]. Moreover, this preventive effect continued up to 199 weeks after randomization. The mechanism proposed was the eradication of latent malignant HCC clones before expansion to clinically detectable tumors.

Neoadjuvant Therapies

The prognostic significance of preoperative TACE still remains controversial. In fact, partial tumor necrosis caused by preoperative TACE might be associated with postoperative disease recurrence, delayed surgery, and increase of liver failure in cirrhotic patients. Therefore, preoperative TACE should only be performed to reduce the tumor bulk for improving the resectability. Liver resection in association with transection of the main portal branch and neoadjuvant or adjuvant locoregional immunochemotherapy could increase the liver resectability, the overall survival, and disease free survival [12]. Preoperative administration of 5-FU and interferon beta may avoid recurrence of coexisting hepatitis B and C virus infections [13].

Future Therapeutic Approaches

As explained above, HCC displays primary resistance to most of chemotherapeutics and this may explain why drug therapies are so unsuccessful. The chemotherapy regimen that has shown the highest response in HCC patients is named PIAF (cisplatin, interferon, doxorubicin, 5-fluorouracil), with a reported 26% response rate and a 9-month median survival [14].

Sorafenib has obtained acceptable results and others multikinase inhibitors (i.e. regorafenib) are in current clinical trials. Another oral multikinase inhibitor is sunitinib, with activity against VEGFR-2, PDGRF a/b, c-KIT, FLT3, and RET tyrosine kinase, that demonstrated no better results when compared to sorafenib [15]. The proposed combination of doxorubicin and sorafenib *versus* doxorubicin alone in patients with advanced HCC has showed improved survival [16]. Another growing area of research is the development of second-line agents for patients who do not tolerate sorafenib or for disease progression despite sorafenib. Several drugs have been tested to target angiogenesis without encouraging results and compared to sorafenib. Bevacizumab (VEGF inhibitor), brivanib (VEGFR2 and FGFR1 inhibitor), linifanib (VEGFR1 and PDGFR inhibitor), ramucirumab (VEGFR2 inhibitor) and AMG386 (Angiopoietin 1 and 2 inhibitor) are only some of the tested angiogenesis inhibitors. Besides angiogenesis, a new possible era may come from the anti-fibrogenic compounds, proposed as novel anticancer drugs, starting with the axiom that fibrosis represents the preneoplastic background. However, to date, no anti-fibrogenic therapy is available. Strategies potentially effective in the treatment of fibrosis should be removal of the initial fibrotic stimulus, targeting activated HSCs, MFBs or liver inflammation and removal or degradation of fibrotic tissue. Removing the causal agent is presumably the most efficient way to prevent liver fibrosis. Because of the complexity and multiplicity of pathways involved in the activation of HSCs, therapeutic targets directed against HSCs are multiple. Anti-TGF-β antibodies, PDGF receptor inhibitors, soluble or truncated receptors and inhibitors of the Smad signaling pathway are currently under investigation. Interferon-β and interferon-γ are shown to inhibit rat HSC proliferation [17] whereas PPAR-γ and its ligand induce reversal of HSCs activation [18]. Also, atorvastatin has shown to induce senescence in activated HSCs and myofibroblasts and could have therapeutic indications in this context. Since the relationship between HSCs and ECM is crucial, pharmacological intervention aimed at targeting this interaction may be a supplemetal tool to prevent liver fibrosis. To this end, the interaction of the soluble Arg-Gly-Asp peptide with the integrin binding site inhibits activation of HSCs and attenuates liver fibrosis in experimental models [19]. Antioxidants including α-tocopherol, resveratrol, silimarin and dimethyl-sulphoxide have been also tested but with contrasting results. Several inhibitors of prolyl-4 hydroxylase (HOE077, S4682), the enzyme that catalyzes the synthesis of the hydroxy-proline residues, critical for stability of the collagen triple helix, have shown efficacy in animal models by decreasing the amount of collagen accumulation [20]. Coexistance of hepatic inflammation and fibrosis represents a hallmark of chronic hepatitis. Several randomized clinical trials of patients with HCV infection treated either with interferon-α alone or in combination with ribavirin have shown stabilization or even a partial decrease in liver fibrosis in repeated liver biopsies. The reduction of the inflammatory reaction, which is often observed by antiviral treatment, undoubtedly plays an important role, but the anti-fibrotic effect of interferon is also beneficial. Several cytokines have been proposed to have an antifibrotic effect. For example, IL-10, an antiinflammatory and antifibrotic cytokine produced by activated HSCs might be efficient in reversing fibrosis. Furhermore, several anti-inflammatory drugs including the cyclooxygenase (COX) inhibitors (i.e. celecoxib) have been proposed as potential anticancer compounds in consideration of the role of inflammatory cells surrounding cancer as an important source of proteases, cytokines and growth factors. For example, antiproliferatives or proapoptotic mechanisms involving the COX-dependent or independent (i.e. via peroxisome proliferator-activated receptor gamma) signaling have been reported [21]. According to the growing body of knowledge about the biological pathways involved in liver cancer, several molecules have been proposed as therapeutic targets. For example, the LPA signaling pathway antagonists including inhibitors of ATX (i.e. PF-8380 or HA130) or an antagonist of LPAR1 and LPAR3 (i.e. Ki16425) seem to be a promising approach. In addition, given the relevant role of LPAR6 in supporting the tumorigenicity of HCC, it is predictable that this LPA receptor could become an important target for developing therapeutic approaches in the near future. A promising therapy is also tivantinib (ARQ197), a selective inhibitor of the MET tyrosine kinase, whose effect depends on the dysregulated expression of c-MET in HCC patients. Another target therapy under development is cabozantinib (XL184), a c-MET/VEGFR-2 inhibitor. As regards the mammalian target of rapamycin (mTOR) signaling pathway, everolimus (RAD001), an inhibitor of mTOR kinase, has been tested in advanced hepatocellular carcinoma after failure of sorafenib (the EVOLVE-1 randomized clinical trial) without promising results. The effects of ERBB1 kinase inhibitors including gefitinib and erlotinib have also been investigated in HCC. For example, in a study by Höpfner and colleaugues, the inhibition of ERBB1 by gefitinib resulted in growth inhibition, cell-cycle arrest and apoptosis in human HCC cell lines [22]. Ongoing studies are now trying to combine molecular therapies, mainly sorafenib in combination with EGFR inhibitors (i.e. erlotinib), mTOR inhibitors (i.e. everolimus), c-MET or IGF inhibitors, and with antiangiogenic therapies. The evidence of estrogen receptors in advanced HCC may justify the use of anti-estrogen therapy in this type of cancer. However, hormones and hormone-regulating agents including tamoxifen, leuprolide, megestrol and sandostatin have been assessed in recent years without encouraging results. Also, immune modulating agents as interferon, thalidomide or activated lymphocytes have been tested without promising results. The combination irinotecan-flavopiridol is another proposed therapy based on the rationale of targeting cell cycle modulators including p53 and p21 protein. The combination irinotecan-flavopiridol is another proposed therapy based on the rationale of targeting cell cycle modulators, including p53 and p21 protein. This combination, particularly suitable for patients with wild-type p53 and with stable levels of p21 has, however, been proved ineffective and poorly tolerated in patients with advanced HCC. Future therapy could be represented by gene therapy aimed at targeting genetic and epigenetic factors. For example, treatment of hepatoma cells with a demethylating agent increases p16 (INK4a) and COX2 expression, and inhibits cell proliferation [23]. Promising preclinical results have been obtained with forced expression of hTERT, the catalytic subunit of the telomerase enzyme, and gene targeting of hepatocyte growth factor (HGF) in an attempt to induce cirrhosis reversion [24-25]. Another therapeutic approach could be transplantation of hepatocytes and bone barrow cells. At present, the most promising cells with potential therapeutic effects seem to be the mesenchymal stem cells (MSCs), as shown by several evidences in animal models. For example, intravenous injection of bone marrow cells, particularly MSCs, appears to have therapeutic efficacy in animals with ongoing hepatic damage, thus contributing to regeneration of damaged hepatocyte mass. Moreover, bone marrow-derived MSC treatment attenuated hepatic fibrosis in rats with thioacetamide-induced fibrosis, raising the possibility of the clinical use of these cells in the treatment of liver cirrhosis.

References

[1] Lim KC, Chow PK, Allen JC, Siddiqui FJ, Chan ES, and Tan SB. 2012. "Systematic review of outcomes of liver resection for early hepatocellular carcinoma within the Milan criteria." *Br J Surg* 99:1622-9. Accessed September 28, 2012. doi:10.1002/bjs.8915.

[2] Jarnagin WR, Gonen M, Fong Y, DeMatteo RP, Ben-Porat L, Little S, Corvera C, Weber S, Blumgart LH. 2002. "Improvement in perioperative outcome after hepatic resection: analysis of 1,803 consecutive cases over the past decade." *Ann Surg* 236:397-406.

[3] Cheung TT, Poon RT, Yuen WK, Chok KS, Jenkins CR, Chan SC, Fan ST, and Lo CM. 2013. "Long-term survival analysis of pure laparoscopic versus open hepatectomy for hepatocellular carcinoma in patients with cirrhosis: a single-center experience." *Ann Surg* 257:506-11. doi: 10.1097/SLA.0b013e31827b947a.

[4] Abulkhir A, Limongelli P, Healey AJ, Damrah O, Tait P, Jackson J, Habib N, Jiao LR. 2008. "Preoperative portal vein embolization for major liver resection: a meta-analysis." *Ann Surg* 247:49-57.

[5] Schnitzbauer AA, Lang SA, Goessmann H, Nadalin S, Baumgart J, Farkas SA, Fichtner-Feigl S, Lorf T, Goralcyk A, Hörbelt R, Kroemer A, Loss M, Rümmele P,Scherer MN, Padberg W, Königsrainer A, Lang H, Obed A, and Schlitt HJ. 2012. "Right portal vein ligation combined with in situ splitting induces rapid left lateral liver lobe hypertrophy enabling 2-staged extended right hepatic resection in small-for-size settings." *Ann Surg* 255:405-14. doi: 10.1097/SLA. 0b013e31824856f5.

[6] Llovet JM, Real MI, Montaña X, Planas R, Coll S, Aponte J, Ayuso C, Sala M, Muchart J, Solà R, Rodés J, Bruix J; Barcelona Liver Cancer Group. 2002. "Arterial embolisation or chemoembolisation versus symptomatic treatment in patients with unresectable hepatocellular carcinoma: a randomised controlled trial." *Lancet* 359:1734-9.

[7] Brian I., Carr. 2014. *Understanding Liver Cancer: A Tale of Two Diseases.* London: Springer Healthcare.

[8] Llovet JM, Ricci S, Mazzaferro V, Hilgard P, Gane E, Blanc JF, de Oliveira AC, Santoro A, Raoul JL, Forner A, Schwartz M, Porta C, Zeuzem S, Bolondi L, Greten TF, Galle PR, Seitz JF, Borbath I, Häussinger D, Giannaris T, Shan M, Moscovici M, Voliotis D, Bruix J, SHARP Investigators Study Group. 2008. "Sorafenib in advanced hepatocellular carcinoma." *N Engl J Med* 359:378-90.

[9] Kubo S, Nishiguchi S, Hirohashi K, Tanaka H, Shuto T, Yamazaki O, Shiomi S, Tamori A, Oka H, Igawa S, Kuroki T, Kinoshita H. 2001. "Effects of long-term postoperative interferon-alpha therapy on intrahepatic recurrence after resection of hepatitis C virus-related hepatocellular carcinoma. A randomized, controlled trial." *Ann Intern Med* 134:963-7.

[10] Arase Y, Ikeda K, Murashima N, Chayama K, Tsubota A, Koida I, Suzuki Y, Saitoh S, Kobayashi M, Kumada H. 1997. "The long term efficacy of glycyrrhizin in chronic hepatitis C patients." *Cancer* 79: 1494-500.

[11] Takai K, Okuno M, Yasuda I, Matsushima-Nishiwaki R, Uematsu T, Tsurumi H, Shiratori Y, Muto Y, Moriwaki H. 2005. "Prevention of second primary tumors by an acyclic retinoid in patients with hepatocellular carcinoma. Updated analysis of the long-term follow-up data." *Intervirology* 48:39-45.

[12] Lygidakis NJ, Sgourakis G, Dedemadi G, Spentzouris N, Kontis A, Nestoridis J. 2000. "Preoperative main portal branch transection combined with liver locoregional transarterial neo and adjuvant immunochemotherapy for patients with hepatocellular carcinoma." *Hepatogastroenterology* 47:1546-54.

[13] Sato Y, Ichida T, Ito S, Hatakeyama K. 2002. "Preoperative administration of 5-FU and interferon beta may prevent recurrence of hepatitis B and C virus." *Am J Gastroenterol* 97:215-6.

[14] Leung TW, Patt YZ, Lau WY, Ho SK, Yu SC, Chan AT, Mok TS, Yeo W, Liew CT, Leung NW, Tang AM, Johnson PJ. 1999. "Complete pathological remission is possible with systemic combination chemotherapy for inoperable hepatocellular carcinoma." *Clin Cancer Res* 5:1676-81.

[15] Cheng AL, Kang YK, Lin DY, Park JW, Kudo M, Qin S, Chung HC, Song X, Xu J, Poggi G, Omata M, Pitman Lowenthal S, Lanzalone S, Yang L, Lechuga MJ, and Raymond E. 2013. "Sunitinib versus sorafenib in advanced hepatocellular cancer: results of a randomized phase III trial." *J Clin Oncol* 31:4067-75. Accessed September 30, 2013. doi: 10.1200/JCO.2012.45.8372.

[16] Abou-Alfa GK, Johnson P, Knox JJ, Capanu M, Davidenko I, Lacava J, Leung T, Gansukh B, and Saltz LB. 2010. "Doxorubicin plus sorafenib vs doxorubicin alone in patients with advanced hepatocellular carcinoma: a randomized trial." *JAMA* 304:2154-60. doi: 10.1001/jama.2010.1672.

[17] Sobesky R, Mathurin P, Charlotte F, Moussalli J, Olivi M, Vidaud M, Ratziu V, Opolon P, Poynard T. 1999. "Modeling the impact of interferon alfa treatment on liver fibrosis progression in chronic hepatitis C: a dynamic view. The Multivirc Group." *Gastroenterology* 116:378-86.

[18] Kon K, Ikejima K, Hirose M, Yoshikawa M, Enomoto N, Kitamura T, Takei Y, Sato N. 2002. "Pioglitazone prevents early-phase hepatic fibrogenesis caused by carbon tetrachloride." *Biochem Biophys Res Commun* 291:55-61.

[19] Iwamoto H, Sakai H, Kotoh K, Nakamuta M, Nawata H. 1999. "Soluble Arg-Gly-Asp peptides reduce collagen accumulation in cultured rat hepatic stellate cells." *Dig Dis Sci* 44:1038-45.

[20] Bickel M, Baringhaus KH, Gerl M, Günzler V, Kanta J, Schmidts L, Stapf M, Tschank G, Weidmann K, Werner U. 1998. "Selective

inhibition of hepatic collagen accumulation in experimental liver fibrosis in rats by a new prolyl 4-hydroxylase inhibitor." *Hepatology* 28:404-11.

[21] Cui W, Yu CH, Hu KQ. 2005. "In vitro and in vivo effects and mechanisms of celecoxib-induced growth inhibition of human hepatocellular carcinoma cells." *Clin Cancer Res* 11:8213-21.

[22] Höpfner M, Sutter AP, Huether A, Schuppan D, Zeitz M, Scherübl H. 2004. "Targeting the epidermal growth factor receptor by gefitinib for treatment of hepatocellular carcinoma." *J Hepatol* 41:1008-16.

[23] Maeta Y, Shiota G, Okano J, Murawaki Y. 2005. "Effect of promoter methylation of the p16 gene on phosphorylation of retinoblastoma gene product and growth of hepatocellular carcinoma cells." *Tumour Biol* 26:300-5.

[24] Rudolph KL, Chang S, Millard M, Schreiber-Agus N, DePinho RA. 2000. "Inhibition of experimental liver cirrhosis in mice by telomerase gene delivery." *Science* 287:1253-8.

[25] Ueki T, Kaneda Y, Tsutsui H, Nakanishi K, Sawa Y, Morishita R, Matsumoto K, Nakamura T, Takahashi H, Okamoto E, Fujimoto J. 1999. "Hepatocyte growth factor gene therapy of liver cirrhosis in rats." *Nat Med* 5:226-30.

Conclusion

The increasing body of knowledge in pathobiology of liver cancer is intended to change the management of HCC in the near future. As discussed above, HCC is becoming one of the most frequent cancers and this is mostly due to emerging metabolic risk factors. Identification of patients exposed to these emerging risk factors will be necessary to introduce specific screening programs, not only in cirrhosis, but also in other emerging conditions such as steatosis/NASH, linked to metabolic syndrome and insuline resistance that would be considered emerging precancerous conditions.

However, currently available serum markers for early diagnosis of HCC have several limitations. Thus, the identification of novel biomarkers is an urgent need. The combination of the new biological indicators of prognosis such as gene expression and molecular signature with the traditional clinical indicators will be of help to accurately predict the patient outcomes and stratify them to identify personalized diagnostical and therapeutical approaches. Another important aspect that must be emphasized here is the crucial role of the tumor microenvironment in HCC development. A better understanding of the cellular functions and molecular pathways involved in fibrogenesis, angiogenesis and inflammation and the crosstalk between these processes and cancer will lead to the identification of new therapeutic targets. It is now clear that targeting not only tumor cells but also the tumor-promoting microenvironment will be more beneficial. Finally, new therapeutic approaches may benefit from the growing knowledges regarding genetic and epigenetic factors as well as metabolic factors related to HCC, hopefully in a more systemic view. What makes more difficult the comprehension of the pathobiology of HCC and the prediction of tumor behavior is the fact that HCC is not a homogeneous tumor, but represents a very heterogeneous collection of tumor cell subtypes. Therefore, further levels of investigation of cellular and molecular profiles may reveal necessary to characterize different subtypes of disease in order to better evaluate and predict cancer behavior as well as to define more effective therapies. The challenge is now to avoid the sanitary emergence that could verify in 2030, as mentioned in the introduction of this book, and gain new insight into the pathobiology of HCC since only a better understanding of the disease will lead to a real positive change in patient outcomes.

Index

A

B

C

D

E

F

G

H

M

N

O

P

R

S

T

U

V

W

Y

Z

α